Howard D. Kurland, M.D.

Illustrations by June Hill Pedigo

BACK PAINS
Quick Relief Without Drugs

SIMON AND SCHUSTER   NEW YORK

Published by Simon and Schuster
A Division of Gulf & Western Corporation
Simon & Schuster Building
Rockefeller Center
1230 Avenue of the Americas
New York, New York 10020

SIMON AND SCHUSTER and colophon are
trademarks of Simon & Schuster
Manufactured in the United States of America
1 2 3 4 5 6 7 8 9 10

Library of Congress Cataloging in Publication Data

Kurland, Howard D
Back pains.

Includes index.
1. Backache. 2. Acupressure. I. Title.
[DNLM: 1. Backache—Therapy—Popular works.
2. Massage—Popular works. WE 720 K96b]
RD768.K87 617'.56 80-24359

ISBN 0-671-41379-1

Contents

Some Introductory Advice

This book contains much wisdom about how to relieve back pains. It may teach you how you can live with back pains without taking drugs. The techniques described in this book can enable you to produce acupuncturelike effects in your own body. You can learn to do so by yourself and without the use of needles or gadgets.

Oriental acupuncturists have achieved pain relief for thousands of years. Studies supported by the United States National Institutes of Health have recently documented the scientific validity of such effects.

When I developed the techniques of auto-acupressure, I did not have the comfort of scientific documentation for such drugless pain relief. However, both personal experience and observation of many patients have convinced me that these techniques are truly effective. You will clearly understand how I personally used these techniques to restore my own functioning when you read about "My Back."

CHAPTER 1

My Back

An eerie premonition of danger haunted me throughout the month. It was the middle 1960s and I was a medical officer in the United States Navy. Attending a medical meeting at the University of California should not have been a menacing thought. Nevertheless, a mysterious sense of dread appeared every time I considered it. When the time of the seminar finally arrived, I overcame my foreboding and drove toward the meeting. I was never able to attend it.

The impact occurred as my car waited at the rear of a line of traffic on a highway in San Francisco. The police report stated that the car which struck me from behind was traveling at 65 miles per hour. My car was sent hurtling on the shoulder of an elevated freeway. The locked-brake skid lasted more than 60 feet. I instinctively clung to the steering wheel, terrified that the car would go over the edge. That encounter with terror remained frozen into my mind for hours afterward. It numbed the awareness of traumatic injuries that my body had suffered.

The morning after the accident, I awoke with my lower back hurting so severely that I could hardly stand up. Sitting was particularly painful. The pain traveled down my right leg. When I tried to walk, I felt a sharp new spear of pain every time I moved that leg forward.

An orthopedic surgeon determined that the car accident had damaged my back. It appeared that there was an injury to one of the discs in the low back area. We will study the intervertebral discs in more detail later, for they are at the root of many of the most intractable back problems. It is enough to say for now that they are pads of tough, resilient tissue that separate the bones of the spine.

For six months I required physical therapy. It included heat treatments, massage, and ultrasonic therapy. After that time, I was able to carry on my normal life again. I had to be careful, of course. My back would hurt sometimes. I had to avoid sitting in soft chairs or in a slumped position. I also had to sleep on a firm mattress at night. But aside from these and a few other precautionary measures, my low back ceased to cause me any significant trouble.

I was not careful enough. Several years after the car accident that started it all, I injured my back again. It happened this time when I was trying to lift a hundred-pound sack of garden fertilizer from the trunk of my car. It was almost impossible to accomplish this feat correctly. There was no way to get my legs under the weight. The design of the car trunk almost required me to lift in a way that put maximum strain on my back. I bent forward, with the car's rear bumper against my knees and thighs. I lifted by pulling with my back muscles alone. Since my back had a previously weakened area, it was prone to injury.

Before I had that sack of fertilizer halfway out of the trunk, a spasm of excruciating pain gripped my lower back and radiated down my right leg. I had injured an intervertebral disc. In the years since the car accident, my back had healed and strengthened enough to withstand ordinary demands. But it had not become strong enough to take that exaggerated abuse.

The injury was significant: I needed complete bed

rest for two weeks. My doctor prescribed painkilling drugs. He also prescribed muscle relaxants to relieve the muscular spasm that is often an important secondary cause of back pain. When I was finally allowed to move about, I had to wear an orthopedic brace. This device was designed, in effect, to take part of my upper-body weight off my spine and rest it on my hips. It was awkward and uncomfortable, but it did allow the healing process to take place. In time, I was able to stand and walk without the brace. My condition improved gradually. I was more careful than before. As long as I was aware of my back's limitations, I found I was able to live a full, active life.

Then, around 1970, I encountered more trouble. It was even more serious. I had been scuba diving with a group off Palancar Reef near Cozumel, Mexico. Returning from a deep dive, more than 100 feet below the surface, we found that the ocean began to grow rougher than we or our diving guides liked. Several less experienced divers panicked in the choppy surf and needed help to board the boat. Struggling to hold my position in an increasingly rough ocean, I had to spend about half an hour waiting to board. By the time my turn came to climb up the ladder, I was utterly exhausted.

My upper body and scuba gear felt weightless in the water. But as I hauled myself up the ladder, all that weight suddenly rested on my spine. As I put my foot on the second rung and started to lift, I felt an indescribably agonizing stab of pain. It was like a high-voltage electric shock going down my right leg.

The orthopedic examination revealed the weakened intervertebral disc had herniated. For medical reasons that are not relevant here, surgery was considered inadvisable. The best my doctor could do was try to return me to near-normal living with my back as it was.

The months that followed were among the least pleasant of my life. I spent the first week under heavy medication, in bed and in traction. When I was finally allowed out of bed, a specialist put me into a formfitting brace that held my back virtually rigid. This brace allowed me to get around, but just barely.

I could walk on a level surface without great pain as long as I moved cautiously, but that was about all. Merely stepping off a low curb caused agony. I could not carry my briefcase; the added weight on one side, even a light weight, put more strain on my injured spine that it could handle. What troubled me most of all was that the injury hampered by ability to work at my profession. I was then, as now, a neurologist. Part of a neurologist's work involves testing patients' muscular strength and responsiveness. To do this, the neurologist must push and pull against the patient in various ways. My injured back would not allow me to do this.

I had to spend many weekends in bed, sometimes in traction. My back needed that much rest if it was going to function at all during the week.

From the beginning, I had tried to avoid taking painkilling drugs because my medical practice required me to be alert. In any case, I did not want to become dependent on drugs, trapped in a life-style of swallowing pills to help me struggle through each day. Instead of getting addicted to drugs, I became addicted to my brace. It was unwieldy and uncomfortable. It made my ribs ache, caused pain and muscle spasm in my shoulders. Nevertheless, I was afraid to walk around without it.

I wore it for more than a year. All during that time, I realized perfectly well what was happening. I knew I was growing more dependent on the brace than was good for me. I knew I would have to get rid of it sometime, somehow, or I might condemn myself to wearing it for life. Now that the healing process was well begun, my back needed a chance to strengthen itself so that it would return to something like its normal functioning.

As long as I wore the brace, no such strengthening could happen.

Yet, I knew there would be a lot of pain when I took the brace off; pain that might last for months, even years. As any backache sufferer knows, this kind of pain cannot be easily shrugged off. How would I carry on my profession and the rest of my life under such conditions? There seemed to be only one answer: to keep myself drugged with painkillers. But that was an answer I had already rejected.

Was there no way out?

I had been casually interested in acupuncture for many years. I had never really studied it or considered it seriously as a bona fide approach to healing or pain relief. Like the majority of Western physicians, I was highly skeptical about its alleged effectiveness. My attitude toward it was one of amused tolerance: it was a type of Oriental mysticism, and if people wanted to play around with it, I did not begrudge them their fun. But if they expected that a visit to an acupuncturist would bring tangible improvements in their medical problems, they were probably wasting their money.

That was what I thought.

A friend in Hong Kong had spent a good deal of time trying to convince me of the merits of acupuncture. During one of my visits with him, as we sailed around Hong Kong's harbor in his boat, he cited case histories of acupuncture patients whose ailments had been successfully treated. Many of these stories were highly dramatic. I might have tried to argue that they were exaggerated or untrue, but I had no reason to think my friend would deliberately try to deceive me. I was willing to grant that the stories might be strictly and literally true. Or at least that my friend was telling the truth as he had seen it, heard it, and interpreted it. Even so, I remained skeptical.

For, as I pointed out to my friend, there could be

more than one way to interpret a situation in which an alleged medical treatment produces an apparent cure of an asserted ailment.

One possibility: the ailment never existed except in the patient's imagination. In this kind of situation, an apparent "cure" might be effected by any procedure the patient believes in, even by a sugar pill, as long as the patient is convinced it is a miracle drug. The procedure or pill might seem to work for this one patient. As far as the patient is concerned, it actually *does* work; but this does not mean it can be expected to work for anybody else.

Another possibility: the ailment was invented by the acupuncturist. This is one of the oldest tricks in the history of medical quackery, and I have never doubted that it is practiced in the Orient as often as in the West. It works like this: a patient goes to a self-styled "doctor" with vague complaints of listlessness, fatigue, loss of sexual vigor, and so on. The doctor convinces the patient that these are symptoms of some serious-sounding disease for which he, the doctor, knows just the treatment. The treatment is, of course, expensive and of years-long duration. It is medically worthless. However, as an adjunct to the treatment, the doctor counsels the patient to improve his diet, get more exercise, stop smoking, and so on. The patient's vigor returns, and he goes away believing he is the beneficiary of a miracle cure.

Another possibility: the ailment was real, but it was already being alleviated by natural processes. The patient would have gotten better whether he visited an acupuncturist or not. He now credits acupuncture for an outcome that was actually brought about by his body's own natural defenses and repair mechanisms.

Thus, as I told my friend, it would take more than a collection of dramatic case stories to convince me that acupuncture was a genuinely useful medical procedure.

Then came the scuba diving episode, the brace, and the drugs. I was desperate for a way out of the dilemma, willing to try anything that offered even the faintest promise. When a chance arose for me to take another trip to the Orient, I resolved to give acupuncture a try.

I had heard many claims for acupuncture, as I have said, not only from my Hong Kong friend but also from other people. Prominent among these claims was the assertion that acupuncture is particularly useful in controlling chronic pain. There are many kinds of pain whose causes, for various reasons, do not lend themselves to a safe, practical treatment. In such situations the indicated procedure is to treat the pain symptom itself. Common types of headache fall into this category, and so do many kinds of backache.

I did not really believe acupuncture could do anything to relieve pain, especially pain as severe as what I was experiencing in my lower back. However, I resolved to keep an open mind on the subject. I traveled to Taipei. With an English-speaking Chinese nurse as interpreter, I visited several acupuncturists, watched their techniques, asked questions. Finally I gathered enough courage to submit to a treatment myself.

The clinic I chose for this first treatment was, like most others I had seen in Taipei, astoundingly dirty. As a Western physician, I had had it drummed into me since my days as a medical student that good medicine starts with conditions of antiseptic cleanliness. Looking around at the acupuncturist's dusty rooms with their grimy, fly-specked walls, I found all my doubts increasing. How could any worthwhile medicine be practiced in an environment like this?

But I stuck with my original decision: I would go through with this one treatment, keep my mind open, and judge the acupuncturist by his final results. If he proved his skill with his needle, I would forgive him for neglecting his broom and scrub bucket.

As I lay down on his dirty treatment table, my back

and leg were throbbing painfully. I had not worn my brace that day. Moreover, the clinic was on the second floor of a building, and the climb up the stairs had thrown my back muscles into spasm. My back hurt quite severely, but I was determined to give the acupuncturist a thorough test.

He inserted needles at several points in my back and shoulders.

And my pain abruptly vanished.

I was astonished. I kept thinking, This can't be true! But it was patently true. My back muscles were comfortably relaxed, and the pain that I should have felt, had quite confidently expected to feel, simply was not there.

That was how I became a student, and eventually a practitioner, of acupuncture. I visited many other acupuncturists in Taiwan, Hong Kong, and Japan; then went on studying the technique when I returned home. Since it is difficult and sometimes unpleasant to insert needles in oneself, I paid particular attention to an alternate technique that the Chinese call *finger needle*. This means using the fingernails or thumbnails instead of a needle. Because I did not have an experienced acupuncturist to treat me, I had to become adept at relieving my back pain by pressing certain body points with my thumbnails. I found that I could alleviate the pain instantly, at the moment a spasm began, by stopping whatever I was doing and applying pressure for a short time. There was no longer any reason to fear the pain. I discarded my brace and my pain medicines.

I went back to the Orient about a year later, hoping to find answers to some questions that had arisen during my studies of acupuncture techniques. I found that many of my acupuncturist friends were excited by *auricular* therapy, the use of needle or pressure points on the ears. It was not a new technique; it was being resurrected after having been ignored for a century or more. It was being grounded in modern anatomy and physiology with innovative work begun by a French neurophysiologist named Nogier. His discoveries were rapidly absorbed in China.

I was enormously skeptical at first. But then I tried it on myself and was amazed by its effectiveness in relieving back pain. Specific areas on the ear, I learned, reflect the entire body in miniature. I developed an ear point system of auto-acupressure. I will teach you how to use both ear point and body point systems to control the pain in your back.

Not long after I returned from that trip to the Orient, I gained firsthand knowledge of the effectiveness of ear point auto-acupressure. I was injured again. An unlicensed fourteen-year-old driver spun his car out of control. I had been riding a bicycle next to a high curb. When the car struck, I was thrown through the air. My back shattered landing on the concrete road. The accident reinjured the same disc that had given me so much trouble before.

After that scuba-diving episode a few years back, I had thought I was experiencing back pain at its worst. I was terribly wrong. The pain at that time had indeed been intense, but it seemed almost trivial to me in the months after the car-and-bike accident. In this latest accident, I had sustained injuries not only to my low back, but also severe injuries to my neck. For weeks, I was in such intense pain that I could not sleep at night without using the drugs which my orthopedist had prescribed.

Perhaps it surprises you that I went back to using drugs, and that I openly admit it in this book. But there is a serious purpose behind this admission. I am a scientist, not a sideshow pitchman. My intent is to tell you precisely what auto-acupressure can and cannot do. I want you to learn how to use it, and develop confidence in its pain-relieving effects. If I were to oversell it, claiming miracles that could never happen, I would only defeat my own purpose.

I kept my intake of all medications to a minimum. While using prescribed pain relievers and muscle relaxants to help me sleep, I took none of those drugs in waking hours. Instead, I used to control the pain and muscle spasm with ear point and body point acupressure. The only medication I took in the daytime was the short course of anti-inflammatory agents my orthopedist advised. (Later in the book I will explain the reason for this, and I will give you some special advice about that particular category of drug.)

Within two months, I was able to stop taking medication for my back altogether. My orthopedic doctor advised me to use both a back brace and a neck brace. However, I was soon able to discard those also. Auto-acupressure, especially ear point auto-acupressure, helped me back to a normal life.

And that is the story of my back. I have told the story to establish my credentials with you. When I talk about pain, I think you will have to grant that I know my subject intimately.

CHAPTER 2

All Our Backs

Back pain, particularly in the lower or lumbar region, is among the most common scourges of mankind. The National Center for Health Statistics says that people visit doctors with this complaint more than with any other, except respiratory infections. Some industrial companies report that back pain is the number one cause of absenteeism: it causes more work time to be lost than does any other kind of ailment, *including* respiratory infections.

Very few people are immune. One commonly accepted estimate is that four out of every five adults, at some time in their lives, will experience backaches that are severe enough to interfere appreciably with normal daily living. Some of these people are relatively lucky: their backaches do not come often or last long. But about a third will find, eventually, that their back pains recur often enough and last long enough to be called chronic.

The human back is a remarkable structure of bone, muscle, ligament, and other tissues. It is strong but often not quite strong enough for the punishment it is required to absorb. As we will see later in the book, some scientists hold that it is innately weak, while others feel it would be strong enough to do its job if the average man and woman treated it with greater care. Whatever the truth of this debate may be, the central fact is that backaches are among humanity's most widespread ailments. No other part of the body's skeletal structure causes trouble so often.

Is there any escape from this suffering? In a very small percentage of cases, breakdowns of the back can be wholly or partially repaired with surgery. But in the vast majority of cases, surgery is not advisable or is not practical. Most backache sufferers must content themselves with trying to control the pain and muscle spasm with drugs.

According to the Food and Drug Administration, more varieties of over-the-counter pills and liniments and other medications are sold for relief of backache than for any other ailment, including headaches and the common cold. There is enormous consumption of analgesics or pain-deadeners. Many are based on aspirin (acetylsalicylic acid), which is produced in this country at a rate of over 15,000 tons a year: up to 50 tons *a day* in some months. For people who cannot take aspirin because of stomach upset or other problems, there are analgesics based on chemicals other than aspirin. Then there are various medicines that claim to relieve backaches by improving the function of the liver, kidneys, bowels, and so on. Malfunctions of these and other organs are thought to cause back pain in some people. Finally there are large numbers of rub-on-the-skin medications. They purportedly alleviate back pain and muscle spasm by producing beneficial heat in the affected area.

In addition to medications such as these, backache sufferers are invited to buy all kinds of gadgetry and hardware. The list is long: trusses, braces, heating pads, orthopedic mattresses, bedboards, electrical massage gadgets, special shoes that allegedly improve the posture, whirlpool baths, and so on.

Some of these nonprescription drugs and gadgets work tolerably well for some people, but they fail to give lasting relief for most. And as we are going to see, even a relatively mild drug such as aspirin can be highly dangerous to certain people when taken over a long span of time.

If the sufferer fails to get relief from over-the-counter drugs and gadgetry, he or she may seek help from a medical doctor. The doctor may prescribe stronger pain-deadening or muscle-relaxing drugs. But these may be even more dangerous than the over-the-counter remedies.

Or perhaps the sufferer goes to a chiropractor. Though the American Medical Association has steadfastly refused to endorse chiropractic as a worthwhile medical technique, it is not my intention in this book to pick a fight with chiropractors. I will only comment that some people say their backs feel better after a chiropractic manipulation, while others say they get only short-term relief or no relief. Forceful manipulation of certain back disorders, which we will discuss in Chapter 5, might result in serious injury to the spinal column, with the possibility of permanent paralysis.

The vast majority of sufferers seem to go through roughly the same history. At first there is a period of desperate experimentation. The sufferer tries all kinds of peculiar medicines, gadgets, treatments, and self-help techniques. Finally, when these fail, he or she falls back on drugs: prescription analgesics and muscle relaxants, over-the-counter remedies, or combinations of these.

In a later chapter, we will examine the potential hazards of such drugs in detail. For the moment let us reflect on some questions:

Do you like the idea of a drug-dominated life? A life in which you must take drugs that dull or distort your intellect? Do you want to take unnecessary drugs? *Especially when you suspect or know those drugs are doing serious damage in your body?*

Until now, most backache sufferers have had to answer those questions in a spirit of unhappy resignation:

"No, I don't like the idea of a drug-taking life-style. I don't like it at all. But what else can I do? It's either the drugs or the pain."

This book offers you a way out of this apparent trap. It is medically sound, effective, safe, inexpensive, and utterly practical.

I call it *auto-acupressure.* In a preceding book, I described the use of this technique in treating headaches. This book details the results of my further studies into the problem of relieving backaches. As you recall from Chapter 1, it is a problem with which I am personally, painfully familiar.

Auto-acupressure is derived from and related to *acupuncture,* an Oriental medical technique in which pain and other problems are treated by inserting and manipulating needles at certain carefully chosen body points. Acupuncture is a technique that demonstrably works (although it has been oversold in this country and has often fallen into the hands of blunderers and quacks). However, a drawback of acupuncture is that it does not lend itself readily to self-treatment.

There are some people who can insert and manipulate acupuncture needles in themselves without qualms, who feel comfortable doing so, and who achieve good results. But they are a tiny minority, and to do so, in my opinion, is dangerous. That is why I developed my system of auto-acupressure. No needles are involved in this technique. You use only your fingers and thumbnails. When you grow efficient with the technique, the results are similar to those that a professional acupuncturist would obtain with a needle.

This book will present everything you need to know to control back pain and muscle spasm with auto-acupressure. I am offering you a double reward that may be among the most valuable you have ever received in your life: *relative freedom from severe and/*

or prolonged back pain, and relative freedom from drugs.

I called it a reward. Properly speaking, a reward is earned. To make the reward your own, you will need to study and learn.

I do not want to mislead you about this. The book you are holding is not a book of mysticism, quackery, or magical-sounding promises. It is a book about honest and thoroughly tested medical techniques, developed by a practicing psychiatrist and neurologist. I will not promise you something for nothing. Before the book ends, I will ask you to do a certain amount of studying and practicing. If you are willing to do that, then the double reward can be yours.

If you are skeptical at this point, I am not greatly concerned. I was profoundly skeptical myself when I first began to consider the use of acupuncture-related techniques in relieving pain. Most of my patients have also been skeptical when I first proposed introducing them to such treatments. But rarely has this skepticism lasted long. I am confident that yours will not last either.

One highly skeptical patient was a man in his seventies. I vividly recall how painfully he shuffled into my office, leaning on a cane, his body bent forward and twisted to one side. He was polite enough to keep his doubts to himself, but after talking with him for a few minutes, I knew perfectly well what he was thinking. His attitude was as plain as the ache in his back: he did not need to say anything about either. He was thinking, Well, I'll try anything . . . but I know it won't work.

I could not blame him for his pessimism. He had been referred to me by an internist, who had given up on him. The internist was the end of a long chain of practitioners who had similarly given up.

The man's ailment, stated as simply as possible, was

a nerve irritation caused by a problem in one of his vertebrae or spinal bones. The problem was considered inoperable because of certain bad risks that were involved. Thus, the man had gone miserably from one practitioner to another, sometimes on referral, sometimes on his own, sometimes as a result of suggestions from friends. When he found no help in the realm of traditional medicine, he went outside it and sought other kinds of help. He visited several chiropractors without getting relief. He started a course of supposedly therapeutic yoga exercises, which made his condition much worse and landed him in bed for weeks. When all these approaches failed, he came back to traditional medicine. When I saw him, he was managing to function by gulping enormous daily quantities of aspirin and prescription medicines.

I told him that I proposed to try acupuncture. He nodded gloomily, obviously not expecting any noteworthy results.

The results, as it turned out, were much more dramatic than I had dared hope. Shortly after I inserted needles in the correct locations, the man stared at me in apparent disbelief. "The pain went away!" he said, in a startled voice. "It just went away!"

When he left my office, he was walking erect. There was only the slightest hint of stiffness in his gait. And he was holding his cane up in the air with both hands.

He told me later that he framed the cane and hung it on a wall of his home as a reminder. In succeeding visits, I taught him what I propose to teach you: how to administer acupuncturelike treatments to yourself, without needles, at any time of day or night and in any situation when a need arises.

Not only did my patient hang up his cane, but he abandoned his pain medications. On my advice, he continued taking anti-inflammatory drugs for a while but eventually was able to do without those as well. On his sixth and last visit to me he shook my hand with unusual warmth.

"You don't know what it's like to have my life back!" he said. "To be able to walk, stand, sit without pain . . . You just don't know!"

As a matter of fact, I did know. There was a time in my life when I, too, was unable to walk, stand, or sit without pain in my back. But I did not tell him that. I just smiled at him and told him I was glad his back pains and his skepticism about auto-acupressure were both successfully treated.

I treated another case of skepticism involving a woman in her late thirties. I will call her Alice R. The primary skeptic in this case was not Alice R., but her surgeon.

She had consulted him because of a severe and aggravated case of herniated disc. This painful condition is often but inaccurately called "slipped disc." We need not go into the medical details here, except to say that the condition involves injury to one of the tough, normally flexible discs that separate the bones of the spinal column.

In many cases, given care and patience, a herniated disc will repair itself to the limited extent that the patient can live a more or less normal life by observing certain precautions. But in more severe cases, surgery is often advised. One surgical approach involves fusing together the bones on either side of the damaged disc, so that there is no longer any possibility of motion in the injured area—and, perhaps, no longer any pain.

Alice R.'s orthopedic specialist wanted her to have this operation. However, he made no attempt to force her or trick her into it. He told her honestly what the trade-offs were. He explained that such an operation unavoidably leaves the spine less flexible than it used to be. Added demands are put on the discs on either side of the fused area. The patient must learn whole new ways of standing, walking, sitting, and lifting.

On the other hand, Alice's surgeon told her, to decline the operation might lead her to much worse trouble. Her damaged disc might repair itself. But, in his judgment, the healing process would take a long, long time. During that time, she could expect to be in serious pain on many days, perhaps most days. The only way to stand the pain, he said, would be to take large and perhaps dangerous doses of drugs.

He told her frankly that he hated to see anybody embark on a program of long-term pill popping. She might easily become dependent on the drugs, even addicted for life. But aside from that possibility, the surgeon was worried about the hazardous side effects of large drug doses.

Balancing all these factors against each other, the doctor felt Alice's best bet would be to undergo the spinal fusion surgery. He admitted it was not an ideal solution to the problem. In his opinion, however, it involved lesser risks than the other course.

One of Alice's women friends had recently consulted me because of chronic, disabling migraine headaches, and I had shown her how to relieve the pain with auto-acupressure. The friend had asked me many questions about the technique, and in the course of one of our talks, I had mentioned that auto-acupressure can also be used against back pain. The friend passed this on to Alice, and Alice now asked her surgeon what he thought about it.

Not unnaturally, he was skeptical. He knew Alice's pain was more than trivial. It was severe enough to require more than moderate doses of powerful prescription pain-deadeners, as well as muscle relaxants. He did not see how any acupuncture-related treatment could prevail against that much pain.

"But I asked him to give me time to try it, anyway," Alice told me as she sat in my office. She sat awkwardly and uncomfortably, her body tipped to one side in a typical backache sufferer's position. "I just want to exhaust all the possibilities before I get on that operating table. My doctor finally said all right." She smiled. "He doubts this treatment will do me any good, but at least, he says, it probably can't do me any harm either."

I nodded. "That is certainly true. That is one of the most important differences between drugs and auto-acupressure. With auto-acupressure, it is impossible to overdose yourself."

As it turned out, she needed only the very lightest of doses. I gave her one acupuncture treatment, using needles in the traditional way. This relieved her pain almost entirely. On a second visit, I taught her how to administer virtually the same treatment to herself, using her thumbnails instead of needles.

And then she went away. I never saw her again. But she wrote a few weeks later to give me a delighted progress report. Her back pain seemed to be entirely under control without analgesic or muscle-relaxant drugs of any kind.

Moreover, her surgery had been called off. I had urged her to visit her orthopedic specialist for regular examinations to make sure that no new damage was occurring in her back. The specialist had already told her this. In the meantime, on the basis of his latest examination, he no longer saw a reason for an immediate operation and felt fairly confident that Alice would never need one at all.

"He says he's sorry he was so skeptical," Alice told me.

But I was in no position to blame him for his doubts. My skepticism, before I began my studies of acupuncture, was every bit as strong as his.

CHAPTER **3**

Why Auto-Acupressure
Relieves Back Pains

A review of recent scientific journals reveals that there are several mechanisms by which acupuncture techniques may produce the relief of pain. Studies commissioned by the United States National Institutes of Health showed that acupuncture points do exist as small areas where the electric charge on the skin is altered. Stimulation of these points can produce physiologic changes.

One study of stimulating acupuncture points with needles and electric current has shown that a certain type of experimentally induced pain was relieved by electro-acupuncture. The relief was equal in effectiveness to a sizable dose of intramuscular narcotic analgesic, such as 10 mg. of morphine sulfate.

The effects of acupuncture in the EEG (electroencephalogram) were found to differ from those associated with hypnosis. In testing the efficacy of acupuncture in relieving experimental pain, *poor* hypnotic responders had as good relief as did *good* hypnotic responders. Therefore, scientists have concluded that hypnosis and acupuncture are separate and distinct methods of treatment. What the scientists produced with acupuncture, we can attempt to duplicate with auto-acupressure.

The beginnings of acupuncture are obscure. There are many legends. One often told story, for which there is no supporting evidence whatever, is that the idea of curing illnesses by needling was developed thousands of years ago in some Oriental war. Soldiers who had been superficially wounded by arrows, so the story goes, noticed that certain long-standing ills and aches were magically alleviated. From there, it was a short intellectual jump to the idea of piercing the skin less painfully and more systematically with needles.

Most such legends are probably fairy tales. Nobody even knows how old a science acupuncture is. What is known to be true is that acupuncture, whatever its roots might be, springs from social, philosophical, and scientific traditions that are quite unlike those we know in the West.

Western medicine has long been oriented toward surgery and drugs. If something goes wrong in the body, we attack it head-on. In a drastic situation, we might remove the affected part surgically. If it seems repairable, we try to repair it. However, we have a third choice. We can treat the ailment and the attendant pain and other discomfort with drugs. This all seems to make perfect sense. It seems so logical that some consider other approaches unthinkable.

In China and other parts of the East, traditional medicine avoided direct confrontation. In part, this was because social and religious customs in many regions forbade the use of cadavers for learning, experimentation, and teaching. In the West, however, scientists were learning by direct observation what a heart looks like and were learning to think of it much as one might think of a mechanical pump. In the Orient, doctors had to content themselves with learning what they could by observing phenomena on the outside of the body. An entire subspecialty of Chinese medicine, for instance, is based on subtle differences in the patient's wrist pulse. It is evaluated, not just by the rate, but by the strength, the "depth," and other qualities that the practitioner feels with his fingertips. Having made a judgment about the "feel" of the pulse, he translates this into a judgment about the health of the heart and other internal organs. He learns all this without actually seeing a heart or examining one physically.

Ancient practitioners of Oriental medicine were not only discouraged from examining cadavers. There were also severe restrictions governing what they could and could not do to the living patient. Women often would not undress for examination or treatment, nor would men of certain social classes. Furthermore, practitioners in some communities were forbidden to spill any of the patient's blood. Sometimes, local customs or religious laws carried no restrictions against minor surgery, such as lancing a boil. However, there always were strong traditions that discouraged any major invasion of the patient's body, such as surgery inside the chest or abdomen.

Thus, one main thrust of traditional Eastern medicine was toward forms of treatment that involved manipulating areas on the outside of the body. Acupuncture is only one of many such methods. Another method that achieved wide popularity in China, for instance, is moxibustion. This is a system in which various ailments are treated by heating certain carefully chosen points on the body. Those points correspond with the points chosen by acupuncturists for insertion of needles.

To the Western mind, such treatment methods seem unnecessarily indirect. This is especially accentuated when the point designated for the acupuncturist's needle (or auto-acupressurist's thumbnail) is on a body area far removed from the site of the ailment. As you will learn later in this book, many of the points designated for relief of backache and spasm are not on the back. Similarly, we have previously presented some points used to relieve headache that are nowhere near the head.

These puzzling qualities of acupuncture and related

treatment systems, that is, the apparent lack of connection between the ailment and the treatment, have contributed heavily to the skepticism that has greeted such treatments in America and Europe. The skeptics' most often asked question is, "If acupuncture works, *how* does it work?"

That is indeed a hard question to deal with. How can I relieve my backache by manipulating various body points with my thumbnails? Precisely what bodily mechanisms act to make the pain go away?

I should begin by saying that the same question is just as hard to answer when applied to aspirin or morphine. Nobody knows all about how these or other pain-deadening drugs work. It is known that they do *some things* to the nervous system and so bring about changes in the perception of pain. But what those *things* are and just how the perception of pain is made to change are still mysteries.

Indeed, nobody is really quite sure what pain is. The study of pain is called dolorology. It is a relatively new medical specialty in Western universities, laboratories, and hospitals. It is new mainly because the subject is so subtle and elusive. Until recently, medical scientists have despaired of making any sense out of it. Often in the past, they tried to explain themselves by proclaiming just the opposite: that the subject is *not* subtle and elusive. "Everybody knows what pain is," they said, "so why study it?"

Trying to support the contention that pain is a simple matter, some scientists advanced the view that there are two kinds of pain, "fast" and "slow." If you accidentally touch a hot frying pan, "fast" pain makes you snatch your fingers away rapidly. An appreciable time later, that first sharp pain is followed by a wave of duller, less intense, "slow" pain. Research seemed to establish that the two kinds of pain are carried by two distinct kinds of nerve fibers running directly from the site of the injury to the brain. It all seemed satisfyingly simple and tidy.

But other students of the subject began to object that there must be more varieties of pain than two. For instance, there is a distinct difference in quality between an "aching" pain and the pain from a cut or stab. Almost everybody recognizes such differences. You can even feel both kinds simultaneously, yet separate them without any difficulty. If your back is aching at any given hour, for example, and if during that hour you happen to walk backward into a sharp-cornered piece of furniture, you can feel the old ache and the new stab at the same time, in the same body area. Such distinctions led researchers to propose more complicated schema of pain categories. In some schema there were four types of pain; in others, there were eight, and so on.

But the subject turned out to be much more complex than that. There are many kinds of bodily sensations that are perceived by some people as painful but by others as something else. Certain types of insect bites, for example, feel like "pain" to one person but "itch" to another. As every dentist knows, some people find that a dental drill always produces pain. Others often describe the sensation as "unpleasant but not actually painful."

To make the topic still more complicated, the same person can react to the same stimulus in different ways. The reaction to pain is in part determined by what else is going on. Every athletic coach is aware of this phenomenon. Football players can get badly cut or bruised during a game. They can even break a finger or lose a tooth without seeming to feel any pain. They go on playing. The pain arrives to surprise them when the game is over.

A physician who served the New York Jets once reported on a conversation he had with an injured man. The man had twisted his elbow joint so badly that he was unable to play for weeks afterward. Nevertheless, he completed the game in which the injury occurred. "It was strange," he admitted to the doctor. "I knew I'd hurt my elbow. I mean, the message got to my brain. It said, Yeah, that elbow is in trouble. But I didn't feel the message as *pain*. The message seemed to say, Don't worry about it till later."

Should that message be classified as a type of pain, or not?

Similarly, a U.S. Army doctor noticed a puzzling phenomenon after a major battle in the Pacific during World War II. The doctor was in charge of a field hospital. Men were brought in with such serious wounds that in many cases, they might have been expected to be groaning in pain. Yet, as the doctor reported later, not all of them appeared to be feeling pain sensations. They conversed cheerfully. Some even seemed to be in a state of euphoria.

Why? Because they had come through the battle alive. Their wounds were tickets that would take them safely home. As one explained with a grin, "Sure, my leg hurts. But I don't hurt."

What message was he receiving from his leg? Should it be called pain, or something else?

Pain is obviously a much more complicated phenomenon than Western students were once taught. What makes it more puzzling still is that pain is often felt at body locations far removed from where one would expect it.

Many back pain sufferers are keenly aware of this. Back problems often lead to a condition loosely referred to as sciatica, or irritation of the sciatic nerve. This may cause the sufferer to feel spears of pain shooting down one leg, sometimes all the way down to the foot. Similarly, people suffering from a heart condition called angina pectoris, which literally translated means "chest pain," often feel pain in the left shoulder or down the left arm, far from the main locus of the problem.

I have studied acupuncture from the viewpoint of modern Western neurology and neurophysiology. My research leads me to think that the effects work somehow through the peripheral, autonomic, and central nervous systems. This is a widely accepted view, for there are many points of agreement between acupuncture and modern neurology. Many acupuncture loci, the points where needles are inserted, are located along nerve pathways with which any Western neurologist is familiar.

What has not been totally elucidated, either by the Chinese or by Westerners, is the exact neural mechanism that produces acupuncture's pain-relieving effects. Some theories state that the nervous system incorporates components called "gates." They operate much like a switch, controlling the passage of pain impulses from the injured site to the brain. When the gates are closed, as in those injured soldiers or football players, little or no perception of pain reaches conscious awareness. Some scientists have suggested that acupuncture works by closing such gates along various nerve pathways.

Another theory deals with a newly discovered group of body chemicals called endorphins. These are peptides that are produced naturally in the brain and that appear to have a powerful opiatelike effect. Some investigators have offered evidence that acupuncture stimulates the brain to release Beta-endorphins, which circulate throughout the body and block or impede pain messages.

The endorphin and gate-control theories are only the latest of many attempts to reconcile acupuncture with Western science. Medical researchers in Europe and America have been studying it since the seventeenth century, when it was first introduced in the West by French Jesuits returning from the Orient. A Dutch physician, Dr. William Ten Rhyne, wrote what is believed to be the first Western medical report on the subject in

1683. Like many other doctors since his time, Ten Rhyne was amazed at some of the effects he had witnessed but confessed that he was at a loss to explain them adequately.

Ten Rhyne concluded that acupuncture must be accepted on an empirical basis. That is, we can observe the effects, and we can produce the same effects again and again, reliably and repeatedly, and so we must trust those effects even though we are not certain about the cause.

Acupuncture undeniably works. Only recently have Western scientists discerned some of the mechanisms that explain *why* or *how* it works. That is undoubtedly a reason why a great deal of controversy has arisen over it. Nor is there agreement on the kinds of ailments against which it is effective. But if I confine my observations to its effectiveness in relieving certain kinds of pain and muscle spasm, I can make the statement unequivocally: *it works*. I know it does because I have seen it work on hundreds of patients and felt it work on myself. American scientists have verified the relief of experimentally induced pain by acupuncture. How useful is it? By utilizing auto-acupressure, you and your back will soon find out for yourselves.

CHAPTER 4

The Structure of Our Backs

Our spines are built of roughly ring-shaped pieces of bone called vertebrae. They rest one on top of another, very much like a tall pile of automobile tires. Each vertebra has a hole in the center (the vertebral foramen), through which the spinal cord passes. There are other openings in the walls of the vertebrae to admit nerves connecting the spinal cord with various parts of the body. Each vertebra has a rearward-projecting knob called a spinous process, to which muscles are attached. Other knobs and projections serve as attachments for the ribs, for ligaments, and for other purposes.

The analogy to a pile of automobile tires is somewhat misleading, mainly for two reasons. In the first place, the vertebrae are not of equal sizes. The smallest are at the top, in the neck region. They grow progressively larger toward the bottom. In the second place, the spine is not straight. It has three major curves: forward at the neck, rearward in the region of the ribs, forward again in the lower back. A pile of tires might be able to stand with three such curves in it, but it would not be very stable. The spine is stable because of the way in which everything is held together.

There are special names for the various parts of the spine. They are:

Cervical: the neck region, consisting of the seven

smallest vertebrae. The topmost of these, and the smallest of all, supports the skull.

Thoracic: the mid-back region, consisting of twelve larger bones. These are the vertebrae to which the ribs are attached. Most people have twelve pairs of ribs. Ten of the pairs curve around to attach to the sternum or breastbone in front, while the two lower pairs are too short to meet in front and so are called "floating" ribs. This arrangement of twelve rib pairs is not the only possible one. Some people have eleven pairs; others, thirteen.

Lumbar: the lower back, consisting of five massive vertebrae. This is the back segment that bears most of the stress in supporting the upper body. Statistically, it is the most likely to suffer breakdowns and cause pain.

The Sacrum: a large bone, shaped something like an arrowhead, that serves to anchor the lower spine to the hips. In a newborn baby, the sacrum consists of five separate vertebrae. They fuse into one massive load-bearing bone in the first years of life. This is the bone that forms the hard rear wall of your pelvic area; you can feel it just above the sharp knob of your tailbone. The part of the hipbone to which the sacrum joins on either side is called the ilium. The joint, hence, is called the sacroiliac—and it is a joint that often gives trouble.

The Coccyx (pronunciation: cox-ix): the tailbone. It consists of four (sometimes three) small vertebrae that usually fuse into one by adulthood. This is one part of the back that rarely gives trouble unless it is injured by a fall or blow. It sometimes becomes painful when ligaments are stretched in childbirth. The coccyx bears no weight. It may be the vestigial remainder of a tail.

These, then, are the bones of the spine: in an adult, twenty-four vertebrae plus the sacrum and coccyx. Now let us see how these twenty-six bones are held together so as to allow us to walk erect.

THE MECHANICS OF THE SPINE

The spine is a compromise between two opposing necessities. One is stability, and the other is flexibility.

Stability: The tall column of bone must be cohesive enough to maintain its essential shape while bearing a heavy weight. It must also withstand both vertical and horizontal stresses. If these twenty-six bones were hinged together as loosely as our elbows, so that each pair of vertebrae could flop back and forth over a 90-degree angle, we would never be able even to rise to a sitting posture. We would certainly be unable to stand up and walk.

Flexibility: The requirement of stability could be met by making the spine a single rigid piece of bone. But that, too, would either make most of our familiar movements impossible or would grossly curtail them. Flexibility is the second necessity. The spinal column must hold its shape—yet at the same time must be capable of bending and twisting.

The way in which nature has fulfilled these conflicting requirements is a masterpiece of engineering. In between each pair of vertebrae is a remarkable structure called an *intervertebral disc*. The disc is made mainly of extremely tough layers of ligament and cartilaginous material. But its central core consists of a softer and somewhat more flexible material called the *nucleus pulposus*.

The intervertebral discs serve several purposes. First, they help hold the spinal bones in proper alignment, one on top of another. (There are also vertical bands of ligament that further stiffen the column and preserve its shape.) Second, the discs act as cushions and separators. They absorb weight and shock. They prevent the spinal bones from grinding against each other. Third, the discs act as limiting hinges. Each disc allows a strictly limited amount of movement between the two bones that it separates. But since there are twenty-six bones, and since each is capable of moving a little in relation to its neighbors, the total amount of possible movement is large.

The spinal column rests on the pelvic girdle at the sacroiliac joint. It is held erect by thick bands of muscle in the back, belly, and buttocks.

CHAPTER **5**

Common Physical Causes of Our Back Pains: A Detailed Overview

Humans are among the longest-lived creatures on earth. During those decades of life, our spines absorb an enormous amount of punishment as we stand, walk, sit, stoop, or lift. At some time in our lives, almost *all* of us will experience pain in the back. It is certainly no cause for surprise that this structure of bones, ligaments, and other tissues is subject to a wide variety of disorders.

This chapter contains a simplified but detailed overview of the common physical causes of our backaches. It is not intended as a complete medical text or as a guide to self-diagnosis. You may wish to study this chapter in its entirety. Alternately, you may utilize this chapter as an abbreviated medical encyclopedia and review only those topics that are directly related to your specific medical problems. If you wish to do so, you will find an alphabetical index at the end of this chapter.

If your pain is chronic or regularly recurrent pain, you should consult a physician. The causes of your pain should be diagnosed. Once you have done that, you should find this chapter useful as a general orientation. When you begin treating yourself with auto-acupressure, I want you to know precisely what you are treating and why.

SIMPLE TRAUMA

This term refers to the most common of all kinds of back disorders. The word *trauma* is a medical term meaning *injury* or *damage*. It does not necessarily mean a visibly serious injury. So it is with the various kinds of simple or mild trauma that can happen to the back. Obviously *something* is wrong, for pain is present. But the most careful examination, including X-ray photographs, may reveal nothing out of the ordinary. Nothing is torn or broken; nothing is out of place. The damage reveals itself only to the person feeling the pain.

There are two kinds of trauma:

Acute: The pain comes on suddenly, resulting from a fall, a blow, an abrupt and awkward lifting motion, a day spent moving furniture, a day spent in a cramped sitting position in a car. The pain is a signal that a ligament, disc, or muscle in the back has been stretched, twisted, compressed, or otherwise forced beyond its normal range of motions. Acute trauma is only one way to describe the condition. It can also be called a strain, a sprain, a wrench, or any of many other terms. As long as it is a simple trauma, with no other complicating factors present, the condition can usually be handled easily enough by a few days or weeks of rest or curtailed activity, plus medication (or auto-acupressure) as needed for pain and muscle spasm.

Chronic: This refers to the kind of hidden damage that can happen to spinal structures slowly over a long span of time. The damage may result from poor standing or sitting posture, from lack of exercise leading to a weakening of abdominal and other muscles that hold the spine erect, and so on. The onset of the pain may be very slow, perhaps starting as a mild "nagging back-ache" that comes and goes over a span of years, gradually growing worse. This condition, too, may turn out to be easily handled. The indicated treatment might consist of exercises to strengthen sagging muscles, better attention to posture, and auto-acupressure to control occasional bouts of pain.

MUSCLE SPASM

This is a condition that can accompany almost any injury to the back (or, for that matter, an injury anywhere in the body). In effect, it is the body's attempt to protect the injured area by preventing movement there. The muscles around the area become rigid, sometimes to such a degree that they act virtually like a hard plaster cast or a metal brace or splint. Indeed, *splinting* is one medical term used to describe the process.

Muscle spasm is undoubtedly useful during the period immediately after an injury. But what often happens is that the uncontrolled muscle contraction continues long after its usefulness has ceased. For example, muscle spasm may last long after the patient is safely installed at bed rest. Then it makes sense to try to stop the spasm. Muscle spasm almost always causes pain of its own, in addition to the pain caused by the original injury.

Not only does the spasm cause pain, but it can sometimes cause damage if it continues long enough. For example, let us say you have a chronic backache caused by the effects of bad posture on the sacroiliac joint. In an attempt to take some load off the traumatized part of the joint, certain groups of muscles might become chronically tense. This pulls the spine into an awkward shape. This chronic tension could be completely unconscious on your part. You do not realize it, but you have begun to carry your body tilted to one side, or tilted backward. In time, the rigid muscles can make permanent changes in the shape of the spine, causing scoliosis, for instance (lateral or sideways curvature), or exaggerations of some of the natural curves.

There are many drugs for relieving muscle spasm, as well as for relieving pain. But as I will show you later, auto-acupressure may accomplish both purposes with considerably less danger from unwanted side effects.

DISC DAMAGE

We are now crossing the borderline from simple or mild trauma to some more complicated and serious kinds of injury. As we have seen, an intervertebral disc may be slightly compressed or twisted. It will usually repair itself without causing its owner severe or lasting pain. But if the damage is more serious—particularly if it is serious enough to be visible to an examining physician—then the prognosis cannot be so casual.

Among the serious kinds of disc damage is a tear in the outer ligament. Still more serious is a tear and accompanying pressure of such violence that part of the nucleus pulposus is forced out through the rent. This is the excruciatingly painful condition called herniated or ruptured disc.

As I remarked in an earlier chapter, the layman's term is *slipped disc*—but it is a misleading term because it conjures up an altogether wrong image of what the injury actually is. There is, in fact, a spinal disorder called *spondylolisthesis,* in which a vertebra actually appears to have slipped out of its proper position. The condition is not uncommon and may cause no trouble. It often turns up by surprise in routine physical examinations of children and teenagers. It may cause problems in middle or old age. However, it has nothing to do with the more common kind of trauma so often called slipped disc. To avoid confusion, I will use the term "herniated disc" from now on.

This kind of disc damage may result from some sudden, violent episode such as a fall or automobile accident. Or it may occur as a result of trying to lift a heavy object, or twisting the body while painting a ceiling. In many cases, a contributing factor may be the chronic trauma we studied before, plus the normal processes of aging. All the body's tissues, including those in the intervertebral discs, grow progressively less elastic after young adulthood. A disc that could take a great deal of abuse at age twenty may tear or herniate under much less abuse at age fifty.

A disc injured in this way can repair itself with proper care. However, once your spine has undergone this kind of damage, you must treat it with new respect for the rest of your life. This does not mean that you must drastically curtail all your physical activities. It does mean that you will need to observe certain precautions (which I will outline later) and that you will probably need to start a course of special exercises to maintain the strength of muscle structures supporting your spine.

In extreme cases, a disc may be so badly torn that there is little or no hope of its repairing itself. A physician may then determine that surgery is the only solution. There are many surgical approaches, including that of removing the destroyed disc and fusing the two neighboring vertebrae together.

RHEUMATISM AND ARTHRITIS

These two words are used, often interchangeably, to describe a bewildering variety of diseases affecting the joints. The words *rheumatism* or *rheumatic disease* usually refer to a systemic (whole-body) disease that may affect the joints or their surrounding tissues. *Ar-*

thritis is a general term used to describe any inflammatory condition affecting a specific joint or group of joints. (Gout is sometimes classified as a kind of arthritis.) However, the distinctions are often vague, and there is no need for us to concern ourselves with the fine points here.

What does concern us is the fact that this large group of diseases can cause, among other problems, back pain. Among the more common diseases in the group are:

Rheumatoid Arthritis: a generalized disease of the body. It attacks women more often than men and is seen most often in people aged twenty to thirty-five, but it can also affect children. The vast majority of people who contract this disease get over it with no serious long-range effects. However, about one person in ten is lastingly afflicted. The disease may start suddenly with a high fever or more slowly with a period of lassitude, aches and pains, loss of appetite. In the more serious cases, it causes irreversible and progressive damage to joint linings, so that the sufferer finds it more and more painful to move the affected joints. In extreme cases, a joint may fuse into a solid mass in which no movement is possible at all.

Ankylosing Spondylitis (also called rheumatoid spondylitis and Marie-Strümpell's disease):   a disease that specifically affects the spine. It is more common in men than women, and it most often begins to manifest itself between the ages of twenty and thirty. The earliest symptom is often a nagging ache in the lumbar region, slowly worsening with time. The ache is caused by abnormal hardening or loss of elasticity in ligaments and other spinal tissues. In many patients, for reasons that are not understood, the progression of the disease stops spontaneously before the trouble is serious. But in others, it may progress until parts of the spine are virtually immobilized. In extreme cases, the entire spine grows rigid from the neck to the sacroiliac—so rigid that the ribs cannot move, and the patient has trouble breathing.

The following five factors are typical discriminators of ankylosing spondylitis: (1) onset of back discomfort before the age of forty years, (2) insidious onset of pain, (3) persistence for more than three months, (4) association with morning stiffness, and (5) improvement with exercise.

Osteoarthritis (also called degenerative or "wear-and-tear" arthritis):   a condition that most often appears in middle or old age. It is characterized by a general wearing away of the cartilaginous tissues that form the bearing surfaces of joints, notably in the spine. Nearly everybody exhibits such joint changes by age fifty or sixty. But in the majority of men and women the changes cause only mild occasional pain and stiffness. In some, however, the changes progress fast enough to cause more serious pain and sometimes crippling stiffness. What happens is that cartilage lining the joints can disintegrate entirely, leaving bone grinding against bone.

Psoriatic Arthritis: the name given to certain arthritic changes that often accompany the skin disease, psoriasis. The skin disease itself is not well understood, but is believed to stem from a possibly inherited error in metabolism. It can be controlled and its symptoms alleviated, but no complete cure has yet been discovered. For reasons that remain largely mysterious, people afflicted with psoriasis have a high incidence of rheumatoid arthritis and other joint diseases.

CONGENITAL DEFECTS

Surprisingly large numbers of people—about half the population, according to one widely accepted estimate—have congenital defects of the spine and its associated structures. In most cases, however, to call them "defects" is something of an exaggeration. They may be nothing more than trivial deviations from the norm. They may cause little or no trouble, and may not be discovered until late in life. The person with such a defect may live a full, long, and active life. However, such defects do, in many cases, cause or contribute to occasional or frequent back pains.

Spina bifida, to take one example, is a condition in which the base of the spine fails to fuse properly—almost as though a piece of bone has been left out. In its severe form, this malformation can cause lifelong total paralysis of the lower body and perhaps early death. However, in a less severe form—called spina bifida occulta, meaning "hidden"—it may cause nothing but the inconvenience of a mild infrequent back pain.

I have already mentioned another such congenital defect, spondylolisthesis, the condition in which a vertebral body is imperfectly aligned with its neighbors. This, too, may go unnoticed until late in life. Then it may begin to cause pain as the surrounding structures succumb to the normal weakening and loss of elasticity that accompany old age.

Another relatively common defect is an abnormal connection or fusion of the sacrum and the fifth (lowest) lumbar vertebra. Depending on the way in which it occurs, this is called either lumbarization of the sacrum or sacralization of the lumbar vertebra. It leads to a certain loss of suppleness in the lower back, but the person with the defect may not experience this as a problem. The stiffness in that area may be wholly or partly compensated for by more than normal flexibility in other parts of the spine. However, the defect may cause back pain under various circumstances, particularly in middle or old age.

DISORDERS OF SPINAL CURVATURE

Scoliosis is an appreciable sideways (or lateral) curvature in the normally straight vertical line of the spine. The deformity may be no more than a temporary disturbance produced by the spinal muscles. Or it may be structural with permanent changes in the bones or soft tissues.

Idiopathic scoliosis is the most important type of structural scoliosis. It is called idiopathic because its cause is unknown. It accounts for 80 to 90 percent of scoliosis cases. It begins in childhood or adolescence and tends to increase progressively until skeletal growth stops.

Lumbar scoliosis may occur to counteract the effect of a sideways tilt in the pelvis. This tilt may occur because the lower limbs are unequal in length or because of deformity at the hip joint.

Sciatic scoliosis is the term sometimes used to describe the deformity resulting from muscle spasm, which we looked at earlier. In sciatic scoliosis, the lumbar part of the spine may list away from the affected side.

Kyphosis is the medical term for an excessive backward curvature of the spinal column. In hunchback, there is an abnormally increased curvature of the thoracic spine as viewed from the side. In the cervical and lumbar regions, where there is normally a forward curvature, any reversal of this constitutes cervical or lumbar kyphosis.

Lordosis is the forward curvature of the spinal column. Normal lordosis is the usual forward curvature in the neck and lumbar regions. However, the term lordosis is commonly used to refer to abnormally increased frontward curvature of the spinal column. Abnormal lordosis is the opposite deformity to kyphosis.

A flat back is one that has a decrease in the normal lumbar lordosis and normal thoracic kyphosis. In hollowback, saddleback, and swayback, there is an exaggerated lordosis of the lumbar spine. In many cases, abnormal lumbar lordosis is caused by poor posture. The condition may also be associated with enlargement of the abdomen, such as may occur with obesity and pregnancy.

TUMORS

There are many, many kinds of tumors or growths that can afflict the spine and its surrounding tissues. They can grow on the bone, in the spinal canal, on nerve tissues, on muscles, on connecting tissues. All of them can cause pain.

Some tumors are benign—meaning that they do not display wild uncontrolled growth and do not threaten to metastasize or "seed" themselves in other parts of the body. A fairly common type of benign tumor is a meningeoma. It is a growth on the tissue around the brain and spinal cord. Another type is a tumor that grows around a nerve root emerging from an opening in a vertebra. Such a tumor is called a neurinoma or schwannoma.

Though benign, such tumors can cause a great deal of trouble and may need to be removed surgically, for example, a tumor that grows inside the spinal canal where the space is rigidly limited. The result could be pressure on nerves or damage to the nerves and their protective tissues. The amount of space inside the spinal canal varies greatly from one person to another. This may become a factor in determining whether a benign tumor is troublesome. In some people, a relatively small tumor can be hazardous. In others with more space in the canal, a larger benign tumor might produce few symptoms or none. In such a case, the physician might decide that surgery would involve greater risk for the patient than simply leaving the tumor alone.

A malignant or cancerous tumor, by contrast, cannot be treated so casually. Such a tumor grows wildly, invades surrounding tissues, and has the frightening property of spreading to distant body sites through the bloodstream or lymphatic system.

Primary spinal bone tumors—that is, cancers which get their start in the vertebral bones—are fortunately not common. But there are many types of cancer that are known to attack the spine, particularly in older people. Among the most feared is multiple myeloma, a tumor of the bone marrow.

More common are the so-called secondary tumors— those that get their start elsewhere in the body and spread to the spinal column. Because of the extremely rich blood supply around the vertebral bodies, such metastatic seeding happens more often than one would wish. Among the more common sites of origin are the breast, prostate, kidneys, lung, and thyroid. A malignant tumor in any of those sites represents a potential threat to the spine.

There are many varieties of malignancy, and they act in many different ways. Some bone tumors will increase the density of the bone they attack, while others will decrease it. All, of course, are dangerous. This is one more excellent reason why anybody with persistent back pain should not merely treat the symptom but should consult a doctor regularly.

Unfortunately, metastatic bone tumors do not always signal their presence promptly. A single standard X-ray examination may not detect anything until as much as one-fourth to one-third of the given bone area has been replaced by tumor. Other kinds of tests can provide an earlier warning. If a doctor examines you on a regular basis, it is likely that he will observe various changes and other clues that will suggest the need for such tests.

FRACTURES AND DISLOCATIONS

Malignancies such as those we have just considered can soften or weaken a vertebra to such an extent that a trivial accident—a mere bump or awkward twisting movement—can break it. When a physician sees a vertebral fracture and learns that it occurred so easily, malignancy is among the first possibilities that will cross his mind.

Fractures can occur in perfectly healthy bone too. The typical spinal break is the compression fracture. It results from a downward crushing force on the spinal column. In healthy bone this most often occurs as a result of violent trauma: an automobile accident, a serious fall, or an attempt to stop a heavy object from falling. At such times, enormous force can be exerted against the vertebral bodies, and one or more of them may crack. The typical compression fracture shows up on X-rays as a wedge-shaped break line, and it is sometimes accompanied by herniation of one or more neighboring discs. It can be agonizingly painful. But as long as there are no complications such as injury to nerve roots or the spinal cord, it usually responds to proper care.

A violent fall or accident may also push a vertebra out of proper alignment instead of breaking it. This might result in a condition called *subluxated facet,* in which one of the vertebra's bony spurs is forced into a faulty position. Sometimes this condition, which is usually very painful, can be relieved by chiropractic techniques or some similar manipulation.

Another possible result of violent trauma is spondylolisthesis—which, as we have seen, can also occur as a congenital malformation. In the typical case, the vertebra slips forward in relation to the two on either side of it. The condition may correct itself in time. On the other hand, it may be severe enough to threaten damage to nerve roots or the spinal cord itself. In such a case, a physician might advise spinal fusion or some other surgery to prevent serious aftereffects.

METABOLIC DISEASES

Many of the disorders under this heading may also be classified under arthritis or rheumatism, those large, loose categories we looked at earlier.

One metabolic disease that frequently causes pain in the back (as well as other joints) is *gout*. Gout is an inherited disease. Because of an inborn error of metabolism, the body produces more uric acid than it can absorb in its normal chemical processes or pass out in urine. The result is that urates, or uric acid salts, are deposited in various parts of the body, including joints of the spine and hips. These chalky deposits, called tophi, can seriously interfere with the mechanical working of the joint, and can cause a great deal of pain and inflammation.

The disease is more common in men than women. It does not often manifest itself before age thirty. In many people, it causes virtually no trouble at all. The high uric acid content may only be discovered during a routine blood test. The urate deposits, if any, may occur in places where they are barely noticed, such as the cartilage of the ears. But in other people, gout can be a crippling disease. Fortunately, it can usually be controlled with proper medication.

Gout is probably more common than most people realize. Indeed, it is likely that many people suffer from its less severe forms without ever realizing they have it. The symptoms may be occasional aching in the back or other joints, and the sufferer may pass it off as a sprain or strain. This in itself may be all right—but problems could arise if the sufferer then takes aspirin for the pain. One of aspirin's chemical side effects is that it can elevate the concentration of uric acid in the blood. Thus, an unaware gout sufferer who swallows a lot of aspirin over a span of years might eventually develop severe symptoms. Auto-acupressure, of course, has no such side effects.

Another metabolic disease that can affect the spine is *osteomalacia*, a softening of bone resulting from disturbances in calcium metabolism. In adults, the disorder resembles rickets in children.

Osteoporosis is another such disorder, but it can develop from any of several causes. It is characterized by a loss of mineral content in the bones and a consequent softening and weakening. It can result from hormonal changes such as menopause or adrenal overactivity (Cushing's syndrome); from long-term fad dieting or other kinds of poor nutrition; or from vascular abnormalities of various kinds.

The typical osteoporosis patient is a woman in postmenopausal years who consults a doctor about low back pain. Her height may have decreased quite markedly in recent years—a common symptom of this disease. X-ray examinations may reveal still another telltale symptom: one or more small fractures in the vertebrae. We noted before that certain tumors can weaken bone to the extent that trivial accidents will break it, and the same is true of osteoporosis. Often, indeed, a patient will not be able to recall *any* specific episode to explain a vertebral fracture. This will immediately suggest to an examining physician that something is seriously wrong with the bone. Osteoporosis will be among the first possible explanations that spring to his mind.

LOCALIZED BONE DISEASES

The diseases we looked at in the preceding section are considered general metabolic diseases. They spring from metabolic errors and omissions affecting the

whole body and may produce their symptoms anywhere in the body. Gout, for instance, can affect any
joint or all joints. Osteomalacia can affect any bone or
all bones. In contrast to these general diseases, there
are some diseases that attack bones in a localized body
area only.

Prominent among these is osteitis deformans, or
Paget's disease. It never attacks all the bones but con-
fines itself to one or a few sites, often including the
spine. The main symptom is a severe disturbance in
the process of new bone formation. In healthy bone,
this process goes on at a measured pace, with old bone
cells dying and new cells continually replacing them.
In Paget's disease, the destruction of old bone becomes
much more rapid than normal. The newly formed bone
that replaces it is not properly constructed. After the
disease has been present for a time, the bone takes on
a peculiar moth-eaten appearance.

Paget's disease and its causes are not well understood. It is particularly baffling because its course can
never be predicted with any confidence. In some patients, its progress will abruptly and mysteriously halt.
In some cases, the disease may resume years later. In
others, the progress is continual but very slow. These
patients may have back pain, but perhaps no major inconvenience until advanced old age. In less lucky patients, the progress is fast. These patients may
experience severe pain and frequent vertebral fractures, and may be crippled at a relatively early age.

INFECTIOUS DISEASES

Some of these diseases, too, are often classified as
varieties of arthritic or rheumatic afflictions. For example, we have already considered rheumatic fever. Flu,
colds, and other common infectious diseases can also
cause inflammation and stiffness in joints. Certain other

diseases such as tuberculosis can produce bone and joint infections.

More common in the United States are pyogenic (pus-forming) infections. Such infections may be either acute (rapidly rising to a climax) or chronic. Acute pyogenic infections of the spine and surrounding tissues often arise from infections elsewhere in the body—typically from the lungs in children, the urinary tract in adults. Fortunately, most such spinal infections respond to treatment quite rapidly if caught in time. With proper care, they usually subside without doing permanent damage to bone or other tissues. However, they can cause considerable pain while they are active.

Chronic infections may be harder to control. For example, one type that is quite common in this country today is chronic pyogenic osteomyelitis, a potentially dangerous and almost always painful bone inflammation. It can get its start from an unclean wound that discharges bacteria and poisons into the bloodstream. The infection may lodge in bones far removed from the original wound. Among the sufferers being seen most frequently by doctors today are drug addicts who have habitually injected themselves with unsterilized needles.

CIRCULATORY DISORDERS

Certain disorders of the circulatory system can mimic sciatica (pain involving the sciatic nerve) and other symptoms of a herniated disc. The patient may feel pain in the lower back, perhaps spreading to one buttock and leg or both. The entire lumbar and hip region may feel stiff; walking or stooping may hurt, and so on. The patient may feel quite certain that the problem is a traumatized disc, when in fact the real cause of the pain is something much more serious.

Circulatory disorders that produce low back pain are

not as common as herniated discs, but they are not rare. I make this point to illustrate, once again, the hazards of self-diagnosis. If your back hurts—and particularly if the pain starts abruptly with no readily apparent reason —you should consult a physician.

One condition that can produce this misleading kind of back pain is *Leriche's syndrome.* This is a clot in the abdominal aorta, a large blood vessel that passes close to the lumbar spine. Another such condition is an *aneurysm* in that same abdominal aorta. An aneurysm is a balloonlike swelling at a point where the walls of a blood vessel have been weakened by disease, a congenital defect, or some other cause. Such a swelling in the abdominal aorta can impinge on one of the lumbar vertebrae or on nerve roots, causing a deep-boring pain.

Statistically, the most likely candidate for this kind of trouble is a man aged fifty or older with a history of arteriosclerosis, or hardening of the arteries. In the recent past, he may have been more than normally troubled by cold feet, and he may also have had several small strokes.

PHYSICAL CAUSES

CHAPTER **6**

Common Emotional Problems That Make Our Backs Painful

Not all back pains necessarily have tangible physical causes. There are many psychological mechanisms that could make the pain seem worse. Psychological causes also could make the pain last months or years longer than can be explained by the physical damage alone. I see such cases often in my work as a psychiatrist. Among the more common:

You-owe-me back pain. Insurance investigators and lawyers who handle accident-compensation cases frequently deal with this phenomenon. Very often, a backache will last until all the legal and financial questions of a compensation case are settled, and then will miraculously disappear.

This sounds more cynical than it is meant to be. True, some backaches are consciously and deliberately faked. But in many other cases, the patient actually does feel the pain. He clings to it, refusing to believe that it is subsiding, because to lose it would be to suffer a financial loss. No amount of testimony by insurance doctors or badgering by lawyers will shake his own belief in the pain. To him, it is perfectly real.

The reason for the backache need not be money. It

could be one of a large number of reasons, such as a need for love. The person with a backache may be saying to friends or family members: You must pay attention to me, and take care of me, because I am in pain. As in the compensation case, this sufferer feels pain because he or she *wants* to feel it. To lose it would be to lose all those special privileges and extra doses of affection that an invalid can command.

I-need-treatment back pain. When a patient consults a doctor about back pain, the real problem could lie elsewhere. The patient might have a sexual problem and might be embarrassed to talk about it. He or she might suspect the presence of some dread disease, may want it diagnosed but may be afraid to mention it.

Again, there is no need to assume the backache is faked. The sufferer may experience real pain. The pain is the body's way of presenting itself for treatment. The patient is telling the doctor, in effect: I am ill, but I want you to discover the real problem by yourself.

The excuse-me back pain. A backache can be made to serve as an explanation for many kinds of failure: in sex and family relationships, in one's career, and so on. The sufferer is saying: Of course my sexual drives are weak. Yours would be too if your back hurt the way mine does. Or: You can't imagine how hard it is to concentrate on work with this kind of constant pain.

The all-purpose cop-out. Backaches, like headaches, can be used to get us out of unpleasant tasks, unwelcome social obligations, and anything else we do not want to do. For instance:

"I'm afraid you'll have to run the meeting without me. My back seems to be acting up again."

"I was planning to invite you out to dinner, but my back . . ."

"I know you're short of volunteers and I'd really like to help, but . . ."

"I was going to spend the weekend cleaning out the cellar, but . . ."

"You know how much I wanted to do it tonight, but my back . . ."

The I-have-emotional-problems back pains. Back pains often turn up as a physical manifestation of emotional pain. A common example is in a typical mid-life crisis. A person arriving at middle age may be seized by a feeling of not having made it in life. He may feel he has not achieved his youthful goals or measured up to some external ideal of success. This very common kind of crisis often gives rise to various kinds of physical problems; they are, in effect, the body's way of expressing that emotional despondency. Frequent or chronic backaches are typical of such unhappy situations.

In many cases, there are tangible physical reasons for low back pain. All are traceable to the emotional problems that are at the root of the crisis. The feelings of inadequacy and depression can lead to harmful changes in the sufferer's personal habits: lack of exercise, sagging posture, loss of appetite, excessive drinking, smoking, and so on. Such changes can undermine a man's or woman's general health and can exacerbate the kinds of chronic back trauma we studied earlier. The result: back pain. Completing the circle, the pain may plunge the sufferer into still deeper emotional despair.

Excuse for drug taking. Many men and women, in the course of treatment for a back disorder, become insidiously dependent on analgesics, muscle relaxants, or tranquilizers. Frequently, multiple drug dependency occurs. They find that they want to continue taking their drugs long after the damaged back has repaired itself and the physical cause of the pain no longer exists. To postpone the feared day when they must abandon their pills, they convince themselves that the pain is still there.

This is not just a problem of the relatively unusual patient who develops a morphine-type addiction to some powerful prescription drug. On the contrary, the problem is widespread. It is quite possible to become psychologically dependent on a mild tranquilizer, an over-the-counter analgesic, or any drug that produces alterations in bodily sensations or moods. The relaxing effects of such a drug may become inextricably woven into the fabric of daily living. The drug makes life's sharp edges less sharp. In time, the patient comes to depend on it as an aid in facing stress and coping with everyday problems. The patient tells himself and other people: "I am taking these pills for an entirely acceptable reason. I must control the pain in my back."

It may also happen that the patient continues taking drugs because of fear that pain will return. As many backache sufferers know only too well, herniated discs and other back disorders can be intensely agonizing. Remembering the pain and understandably fearing it, the sufferer may go on swallowing analgesics and other drugs long after the physical pain has left. This person can very easily convince himself or herself that the dreaded pain is lurking down there as before: that the pain is waiting to return at the first sign of a lapse in vigilant pill popping. "I can feel the pain beginning to build up whenever a pill starts to wear off," the patient insists. It is often hard for a doctor or anyone else to convince such a patient that the feared back pain may only be a fear. These patients are so certain the pain exists that in their minds it does.

CHAPTER **7**

Listening to Our Doctors Talk About Our Backs

The previous chapters have not attempted to cover every conceivable cause of back pain, but rather to give you some brief insights into the complexity of the subject. Your own back pains may have many causes, some physical, some emotional. Identifying them and sorting them out is a task for your physician. But it is likely that you can help him in making the diagnosis and choice of treatment. Later you can be an effective participant in that treatment, if you have an informal layman's knowledge of the spine and the many problems it may encounter. That is why I believe you will find this chapter useful.

In talking about your particular case, your physician may use different terms and phrases than I have used. It is also likely that your well-meaning friends, neighbors, and family members will attempt to make laymen's spot diagnoses of your problem. They may confuse you with still other terms, slipped disc, for instance. Back disorders are so common that it often seems as if a separate language has grown up around them. In order to understand your own problem, here is a very brief glossary of the more common terms that a backache victim is likely to hear in and out of a doctor's office:

Nonarticular Rheumatism. This is a medical term

encompassing all those diseases and conditions that involve the soft tissues around joints, but do not directly involve the joints themselves. The most common types of nonarticular rheumatism are grouped under another medical term: fibrositis.

Fibrositis.   This, again, is not the name of a specific condition but is a catch-all word. It refers to painful, inflammatory conditions involving ligaments, muscles, muscle tendons, and so on. The simple trauma we looked at earlier might often be classed as a variety of fibrositis. Or the inflammation and other problems might occur because of some systemic infection such as influenza or the common cold.

Lumbago.   This is more a layman's term than a medical one. It means any undiagnosed pain in the lumbar region, the small of the back. There is no specific disease called "lumbago." At one time, medical authorities did use the word to describe what they thought was a specific condition, but that was in a day when little was known about spinal disorders such as gout or the herniated disc. Now that it is possible to name such disorders more specifically, "lumbago" has more or less passed out of usage.

Sciatica.   This is the name of a symptom, not a disease. In many back disorders, but especially in cases of disc injury, roots of the sciatic nerve get irritated. The sciatic nerve is a great bundle of nerve fibers, the longest in the body, with its roots in the lower back. (Its name means "hip joint nerve.") The nerve splits into two main pathways and goes through the buttock muscles and down the legs into the feet. When the roots in the lumbar region are irritated, the sufferer may feel "referred" pain in one buttock and leg, sometimes in both. The pain may go clear down to the foot. In about 70 percent of cases, it is accompanied by sensations of numbness or weakness in the legs, knees, or ankles. Often the sufferer finds it hard to move the straightened leg forward for more than a few inches. Unless the pain is caused by disease or injury directly involving the sciatic nerve itself, the condition usually subsides as the back injury repairs itself.

If you suffer back pains from a disorder not mentioned in this brief chapter, please refer to the appropriate section in the previous two chapters. In Chapters 5 and 6, there is a more detailed discussion of the common physical and emotional causes of back pains. All the conditions listed in Chapters 5, 6, and 7 can be associated with pain and muscle spasm. Now let us look at the drugs that backache sufferers may take for these problems and others. As you will see, many of the commonly used drugs are quite dangerous. In my opinion, not all of them are always necessary.

8

Drugs for Our Back Pains: A Reference Source

Correctly applied, auto-acupressure has no dangerous side effects. When you use it as I advise, you cannot "overdose" yourself with it. When the effect of one application wears off, you can safely give yourself another treatment, no matter how much or little time has elapsed. You can use it heavily or lightly, regularly or intermittently, for as many months or years as the need persists. It cannot poison you.

None of this is true of drugs. Almost all the medicines used against back pains have unwanted side effects. That includes drugs which are considered mild enough to be sold without prescription. Side effects range from the unpleasant to the potentially fatal.

If you are a back pain sufferer, it is likely that you have been taking medication of some kind: prescription medicines, over-the-counter drugs, or both. Perhaps you have taken a great deal of medication. Many back pain victims do. As a back pain sufferer myself, I am well aware of the temptation to indulge in excess medication. It is especially great on those days when the pain makes coping practically impossible.

Even if your intake of drugs has been moderate, you may have noticed certain side effects. You may have worried about the possibility of others. Some side effects occur promptly and are readily apparent: dizziness, lethargy, skin rash, and so on. Other side effects are hidden. They sometimes take place slowly over a span of years, perhaps insidiously damaging some vital organs beyond repair.

In this chapter, I am going to list drugs that are most often prescribed for and used by people suffering from common back disorders. Having listed the drugs and briefly described their uses, I will describe their known side effects. The chapter is not intended as a manual of pharmacology, but as a layman's quick guide. In all likelihood, you will find listed here one or more medications that you have been taking. If you want to refer to your own medications quickly, you will find an alphabetical index of drug names at the end of the chapter.

As you will see, many of the side effects of these drugs are not trivial. If you have been worried about them, your worry is entirely reasonable.

Am I counseling, therefore, that you abandon your medicines? Absolutely *not*. Many back disorders require strong medication, and the unwanted side effects must be accepted as part of the condition. The decisions to reduce or discontinue a prescribed drug should never be made without consulting your physician.

What I do counsel is that, with your doctor's concurrence, you try using auto-acupressure to control pain and muscle spasm. If you find that it works for you, then it may be possible to cut down your use of certain medicines. Perhaps you will be able to do away with some drugs entirely.

Your physician may feel that certain other drugs are essential to your therapy. He may want you to continue taking them. By all means do so.

If you can eliminate any unnecessary medication with which your body must contend, you will have won a major battle.

Perhaps, indeed, you will have won a longer and healthier life.

1. DRUGS PRESCRIBED FOR MUSCLE SPASM

Centrally Acting Skeletal Muscle Relaxants

This is a rather vaguely defined group of drugs. It includes many medicines that are more commonly thought of as sedatives, tranquilizers, antianxiety or antitension agents. Skeletal muscle relaxants might not have a selective muscle-relaxing action in man that is separate from their sedative effects. As a matter of fact, some of these drugs are sometimes promoted as primarily muscle relaxants, and at other times as primarily sedatives or tranquilizers. It is as though the manufacturers themselves are not quite sure what are the primary effects of these drugs or how they should be used.

A doctor prescribes relaxants in an attempt to relieve the muscle spasm that often accompanies disorders of the back. As we saw in the last chapter, prolonged muscle spasm may interfere with the body's natural repair processes. At the very least, such spasm usually produces pain. Thus, there is no question that it is a good idea to relax the affected muscle groups when possible. The question is: which treatment does the job best?

Those who prefer the use of drugs have a wide variety to choose from. Among the most commonly prescribed skeletal muscle relaxants are these:

> carisoprodol (trade names: Rela, Soma)
> chlorzoxazone (Paraflex)
> methocarbamol (Robaxin)
> orphenadrine citrate (Norflex)
> cyclobenzaprine (Flexeril)

Antianxiety Agents Prescribed for Muscle Spasm

There are many antianxiety drugs that are similar in chemical structure to those listed as muscle relaxants.

As I mentioned, such drugs are often prescribed inter-changeably for the two purposes.

The action of barbiturates and other sedatives on muscle spasm is not clearly understood. We do not know whether they work through a direct muscle-relaxing effect or indirectly through general sedation. In animal experiments, large intravenous doses of certain of these drugs do seem to reduce many spinal reflexes. But there is no clear evidence that the same effects happen in man, especially not with the usual recommended oral doses. Such drugs sometimes bring temporary relief from pain. However, there is no trustworthy evidence that they help bring about any objective improvement in chronic back disorders; therefore, they are not indicated for the long-term management of chronic disorders.

Among antianxiety medicines most often prescribed for muscle spasm are:

chlordiazepoxide (trade name: Librium)
diazepam (Valium)
meprobamate (Equanil, Miltown)

Side Effects and Hazards

One difficulty with all muscle relaxants is that they can interfere with normal activity. If you take such drugs while confined to bed, they can be very comforting. But for the patient who wants to go about his or her daily work, muscle relaxants unavoidably cause a troublesome general weakness. This weakness may be little more than a nuisance, leading to unsteadiness on the feet or an annoying sense of fatigue. Or it can be much more serious. By weakening abdominal and back muscles that normally help support the spine and the upper body, back disorders may become prolonged or more severe.

With or without this muscle-weakening effect, barbiturates and other tranquilizers prescribed for muscle spasm can influence judgment, physical coordination, and general alertness. People taking such drugs should be extremely cautious about driving cars and operating other potentially dangerous machinery.

It is hard to formulate rules about the effects of tranquilizers and muscle relaxants. Dosages differ, and people also differ in their reactions to a given dosage. Some men and women seem able to take moderate doses of such drugs without undergoing marked changes. But in other people, even a relatively small dose can cause such drastic impairment of normal abilities that they absolutely should *not* get behind the wheel of a car. If you are in this latter group, and if you depend on a car for commuting, shopping or other activities, a back disorder could bring you up against a difficult choice. Either you must try to bear the pain, or you must take drugs and live with serious restrictions on your life.

Another hazard of tranquilizers is that long and continued use can lead to psychic or physical dependence. Abrupt discontinuance can bring on severe withdrawal symptoms. People using large amounts of meprobamate over a prolonged period have been known to suffer epileptic seizures when they abruptly stopped taking the drug.

Large oral doses of either tranquilizers or the primary muscle relaxants have been known to cause a variety of other problems. Among them are nausea, vomiting, constipation, diarrhea, respiratory depression (extremely dangerous for people with emphysema and other diseases of the lungs and respiratory tract), fast heartbeat, and low blood pressure. These side effects do not occur often, but they are definite potential hazards.

Even relatively small doses of tranquilizers and muscle relaxants can cause drowsiness, dizziness, blurred vision, and allergic reactions such as rash and itching. Sometimes—as is true of nearly all drugs—an unexpected allergic reaction can be violent and dangerous. This happens rarely, but the danger does exist.

All these hazards become more troublesome in the case of a pregnant woman. Medical science does not yet know nearly enough about what happens in the womb when a mother takes drugs of various kinds. Until we learn more, caution is advisable. If a drug produces unwanted effects in an adult, there is a clear possibility that it will produce those same effects in a fetus. Moreover, the use of some of these drugs during pregnancy is related to an increased incidence of birth defects.

2. DRUGS PRESCRIBED FOR PAIN

Strong Analgesics

Analgesics, or pain-relieving drugs, are generally divided into two groups: strong and mild. The strong ones are intended to relieve the more severe kinds of pain, including the pain that sometimes accompanies back disorders.

As we noted in a previous chapter, pain is an extremely complex phenomenon. The perception of pain differs from patient to patient, and also from time to time in the same patient. People's reactions are particularly hard to predict in the case of severe pain. That is why nearly all strong analgesics are formulated to attack pain in at least two distinct ways. First, they act to raise the threshold of pain perception. Second, they act to suppress the patient's anxiety, depression, and other emotional factors that might be intensifying the subjective pain sensation.

Almost always, strong analgesics cause some alteration of consciousness, or behavior, or both. It would be nearly impossible to effect strong pain without causing such changes.

The strong analgesics are classified into two types: narcotic and non-narcotic.

Narcotic analgesics can be subdivided into four classifications:

1. opium preparations
2. purified alkaloids of opium, such as morphine
3. semisynthetic modifications of morphine, such as Numorphan, Dilaudid, and oxycodone (which is the narcotic in the combination drugs sold under the trade names of Percodan, Tylox and Percocet-S)
4. synthetic morphinelike compounds

In this last classification—the synthetic morphinelike compounds—we can group drugs by chemical structure. Among them are: phenylpiperidine derivatives, such as meperidine (Demerol); morphinan or phenanthrene derivatives, such as levorphanol (Levo-Dromoran); butorphanol tartrate (Stadol), a dihydroxymorphinan narcotic antagonist analgesic; diphenylheptane derivatives, such as methadone (Dolophine); propionanilide derivatives, such as Fentanyl or Sublimaze.

Non-narcotic analgesics, so-called because they are not subject to government regulations dealing with narcotic control, fall into two main groups:

1. phenothiazine derivatives, such as methotrimeprazine (Levoprome)
2. benzomorphan derivatives, such as pentazocine (Talwin)

Side Effects and Hazards

Since the strong analgesics alter patients' consciousness and moods, sometimes very powerfully, it might be expected that addiction would be a potential problem. It is. Though the majority of patients are able to stop taking these drugs without great difficulty, there are some who develop a strong dependency. The like-lihood of dependency is less with non-narcotic analge-sics, but there is always a risk. Doctors worry about administering *any* strong analgesic to patients with a known history of drug abuse.

That difficulty is complicated by the problem of tol-erance. Some patients demand increasing amounts of these drugs as time goes by. The physician must then ask a question to which there may be no ready answer: is the patient asking for more analgesic because the pain is actually growing more severe, or because more of the drug is necessary to accomplish the same result? This development of tolerance—in which the patient needs increasing doses to get the physical and/or mood-changing effects he craves—is often among the early warning signs of a growing dependency.

The doctor is torn by conflicting motives: his wish to relieve the patient's pain and his fear of overdosing or creating addiction. This is an unavoidable problem with all strong analgesics. It is a problem that does not exist in the case of auto-acupressure.

Another highly troublesome problem with strong an-algesics—perhaps the worst danger of all—is their ten-dency to cause changes in respiratory functions. The result can be a dangerous decrease in ventilation. If this condition goes unattended for a long enough time, the lack of sufficient oxygen can cause irreversible damage to the brain. Thus, it is a standard precaution to have oxygen handy when a patient is being given such drugs for the first time. The danger is especially grave, of course, in the case of patients with bronchitis, chronic obstructive pulmonary disease (emphysema), or other respiratory disorders.

Like the muscle relaxants and tranquilizers that we looked at previously, strong analgesics may also inter-fere with a patient's daily living. Indeed, they may virtually slow it to a standstill. These drugs cause drowsiness and clouding of the intellect. There is often a general deterioration of the mental and physical capacities that the patient would command when fully alert and undrugged. This might cause no problem if the patient is lying in bed. It might be considered just a passing nuisance if the drugs are to be administered for only a week or so. But the drugs might present serious difficulties if the patient must take such drugs over a long span of time, and if he or she wants to continue with work and family responsibilities. Some men and women are so powerfully affected by strong analgesics that they cannot even perform seemingly simple tasks requiring only a moderate degree of concentration and coordination.

Among other unwanted side effects of these drugs are cardiovascular effects, such as a slowing of the heartbeat and a drop in blood pressure. There might be various difficulties in the urinary tract, including muscular spasms, painful urination, and sometimes acute urine retention. Also, there might be an assortment of digestive upsets, including nausea and constipation. Less commonly, such drugs can produce allergic reactions such as itching, rash, or (rarely) acute shocklike states.

Mild Analgesics

These drugs are prescribed for relief of mild to moderate pain. Even in large doses, they are not very effective against severe pain.

They are generally divided into two groups: first, those related chemically to the strong analgesics; and second, the analgesic-antipyretics, or antifever agents. There is also a third large group: trade-named drugs that are combinations of two or more different agents and purportedly accomplish two or more different purposes. Let us consider the three groups separately.

Drugs Related to Strong Analgesics

Three of the best-known and most commonly used of these drugs are codeine, propoxyphene (sold under the trade names Darvon, Dolene, SK-65, and Darvon-N), and ethoheptazine (Zactane).

Codeine is a narcotic, though a mild one. It is about twenty times as strong as aspirin on a weight-for-weight basis. A half-grain has roughly the same pain-relieving effect as 10 grains, or two standard-sized tablets, of aspirin. As a narcotic, it is of course potentially addictive; it is especially so when codeine is prescribed in conjunction with sedatives or antianxiety agents. However, the risk of dependency is not considered unacceptably high when the drug is given in small oral doses.

Propoxyphene, more commonly known as Darvon, is chemically related to methadone (Dolophine). It has about half to two-thirds the weight-for-weight potency of codeine. Darvon-N is about two-thirds the potency of an equivalent weight of Darvon. Propoxyphene is also potentially habit forming; it is less so than codeine but more so than aspirin. Another disadvantage is that it has less powerful antifever and anti-inflammatory effects than aspirin. For this reason it is often prescribed in conjunction with aspirin. As with codeine, the additive effects of the combination of drugs increase the potential hazards.

Ethoheptazine, sold under the trade name Zactane, is chemically related to Demerol. It is promoted for relief of mild to moderate pain. It appears to have roughly the same analgesic effect as aspirin, but clinical studies of its pain-relieving potency have not been conclusive. It has no anti-inflammatory or antifever effects. Its adverse effects are principally stomach distress, dizziness, and itching. The adverse effects, like the beneficial effects, appear to be quite mild.

The Analgesic-Antipyretics

These are divided into several classes:

Salicylates, of which the most widely used and best known is aspirin. Aspirin was once a trade name, owned by the Bayer Company, but it lost its legal protection and is now considered a generic word that need not be dignified with a capital initial. The drug is most familiar under this generic name, but it is also sold under the trade names A.S.A., Ecotrin (enteric-coated aspirin) and Measurin (timed-release aspirin).

Aspirin is a principal ingredient in approximately 50,000 nonprescription drugs. The following is a list of some of the most familiar trade names:

Anacin
Arthritis Strength Bufferin
Bufferin
Cope
Empirin
Excedrin
Vanquish

Aspirin is the prototype of this analgesic-antipyretic group. It is considered by many to be the drug of choice when a mild analgesic is called for, despite some potentially serious side effects. We will look at those side effects later.

For patients who cannot safely take aspirin for one reason or another, other salicylates may be prescribed. One is sodium salicylate, usually sold under its generic name. It appears to have somewhat less effect than aspirin on a weight-for-weight basis. Its advantage is that it lacks some of aspirin's dangerous side effects. In particular, it causes less irritation and bleeding in the stomach. A disadvantage is that it cannot be taken by people on a low sodium (salt) diet.

Another such drug is salicylamide, sold under the

trade names Amid-Sal, Salamid, and Salrin. It appears to have fewer adverse effects than aspirin, but there have been no controlled studies involving doses of comparable strength. Still another is magnesium salicylate (Magan).

Phenacetin is another mild analgesic-antipyretic in fairly common use. It is chemically related to an older drug, acetanilide, which it has largely replaced. It has roughly the same analgesic and antifever effects as aspirin, but it has little or no anti-inflammatory action. It is often prescribed for patients with gout. Unlike aspirin, it does not counteract the effects of certain gout medicines.

This drug is often used in combination with other drugs. In combination with aspirin and caffeine, phenacetin is sold under the familiar initials A.P.C. and with the trade name of Empirin.

Para-aminophenol derivatives, such as acetaminophen, which is sold under the trade names Tylenol and Datril. Aspirin Free Anacin 3 contains acetaminophen and caffeine. This drug has roughly the same pain-relieving and antifever effect as aspirin (though its action differs from one patient to another). It does not have so strong an anti-inflammatory effect. Its major advantage is that it usually is not as irritating to the gastric lining as aspirin. It is often recommended for patients who have gastric ulcers or gout. It is also used for patients who are on anticoagulants or have other disorders that would make aspirin unsafe for them.

Aspirin and acetaminophen combination drugs. This is a relatively new but fast-growing group of non-prescription drugs. These combination drugs have the potential side effects and hazards of both drugs. Some familiar trade names are:

Excedrin
Excedrin P.M.
Vanquish

Pyrazolone derivatives such as dipyrone, trade-named Narone and Pyrilgin, are not used routinely because of some potentially dangerous side effects. These drugs are prescribed only when there is some pressing reason not to use other mild analgesics.

Newer drugs that are not related chemically to any of the others in this group. Among these is indomethacin, or Indocin. This is an analgesic with roughly the same pain-relieving, antipyretic and anti-inflammatory effects as aspirin. However, because of some fairly serious adverse effects, it is generally recommended only in special cases—gouty arthritis and rheumatic disorders are examples—when, for various reasons, other analgesics would cause still worse problems.

Combination Drugs

These are all trade-named drugs in which analgesics are mixed with various other agents. In almost all these cases, the rationale for mixing drugs in this way is questionable. One might ask what is gained by mixing two commonly available drugs. A physician could easily prescribe them separately and have greater control over the relative amounts. Some doctors question the value of these combination drugs because the amount of a given ingredient present in the mixture seems too small to have much beneficial effect.

Here are some of the most familiar combinations:

- Combinations in which a mild analgesic is mixed with a stronger one, narcotic or non-narcotic. Familiar trade names:

  Meperidine and Dem-A.P.A.P. (Demerol mixed with A.P.C.)
  Percodan (oxycodone and A.P.C.)
  Percocet-5 (oxycodone and acetaminophen)
  Talwin (pentazocine and aspirin)
  Tylox (oxycodone and acetaminophen)

• Mixtures containing a mild analgesic and a sedative. Familiar trade names:

Equagesic
Fiorinal
Fiorinal with codeine
Norgesic
Parafon Forte
Percogesic
Percogesic with codeine
Phenaphen
Phenaphen with codeine
Robaxisol
Soma Compound
Soma Compound with codeine

• Combinations containing codeine, in addition to those just listed. Familiar trade names:

Ascodeen-30
Ascriptin with codeine
Empirin Compound with codeine phosphate (available in several different formulations)
P-A-C Compound with codeine sulphate
Tylenol with codeine (also available in several formulations)

• Combinations containing propoxyphene. Familiar trade names:

Darvon with A.S.A.
Darvon-N with A.S.A.
Darvon Compound
Darvocet-N
Dolene Compound 65
SK-65
Wygesic

• Mixtures containing ethoheptazine. Familiar trade names:

Zactirin
Zactirin Compound-100

- Compounds of aspirin and antacids. Familiar trade names:

  Alka-Seltzer
  Ascriptin
  Bufferin

These drugs are referred to generically as buffered aspirin because the antacid is supposed to act as a buffer against aspirin's potentially harmful effects in the gastrointestinal tract. However, in most such products the amount of antacid is too small to have much if any effect. Controlled studies have failed to show that the claimed buffering action significantly reduces the hazards of taking such drugs over a long period, as against the hazards of taking plain aspirin.

Some nonprescription mixtures of aspirin are effervescent tablets; when dissolved they become highly buffered solutions of sodium acetylsalicylate. Such preparations may cause less stomach irritation and produce faster passage into the circulatory system. However, taken in large doses or with repeated use, the absorbable antacid in these preparations may make the urine alkaline: that results in decreased salicylate blood levels because of more rapid elimination through the kidneys.

Side Effects and Hazards

Aspirin, or acetylsalicylic acid, is the most common analgesic. It is often considered the drug of choice in many circumstances. The Bayer Company, former owner of the Aspirin trade name, has recently been publishing ads in which a physician is quoted as saying: "Aspirin is undoubtedly the safest pharmaceutical known to modern medicine." It is indeed a valuable drug: cheap, effective against mild pain, inflammation, and fever. It is useful in all kinds of therapeutic situations and considered mild enough to be sold freely without governmental red tape. Bayer has a right to be proud of it. What the company's ads do not say, however, is that this seemingly innocuous drug can cause a long list of unwanted effects and can even be fatal.

Aspirin is the leading cause of drug-poisoning deaths in children. It is the second leading cause of drug-overdose deaths of adults in the United States. Some of these are accidental deaths of children. Other deaths are intentional adult suicides. Still others are accidental overdoses by adults, who were apparently not aware how toxic this drug can be when one exceeds the normal recommended dosage limits.

Such single-overdose deaths are dramatic and sometimes make local newspaper headlines. Slower deaths make headlines less frequently. In many people, aspirin irritates the delicate inner lining of the stomach and causes a condition that physicians call *occult* (hidden) bleeding. Sometimes as much as a teaspoon of blood can be lost after a normal 10-grain dose (two standard tablets). This can lead to very serious problems if it continues long enough. It can exacerbate ulcers and other stomach disorders. It can cause ulcerations where none existed before. In time, this condition may be fatal.

Aspirin can contribute to or exacerbate iron-deficiency anemia if taken over a long span of time. Because of the effect of aspirin on a type of blood cell called platelets, blood-clotting time is increased. Therefore it cannot be used safely by patients with bleeding disorders of various kinds. It can be toxic to the liver and thus may not be safe for people with liver disorders. It may also be harmful to patients with diabetes, for under some circumstances it can dangerously enhance the effects of certain antidiabetic medications.

There is also evidence that aspirin can cause trouble for pregnant women. According to one medical study, women who are regular heavy users of aspirin tend to have more difficult pregnancies, more complications in delivery, and more abnormal births.

Long-term heavy use or overdosing of aspirin can also lead to a group of disorders loosely grouped under the name *salicylism*, or aspirin poisoning. Among the earliest signs are tinnitus (ringing or other noises in the ear) and hyperventilation (fast, heavy breathing). Children develop aspirin-induced hyperventilation more rapidly than adults. Salicylism may cause dizziness, lethargy, and confused states. Paradoxically, it may produce headaches. There may also be various allergic reactions: itching, skin rash, or asthmalike shock reactions.

Acetaminophen (Tylenol, Datril) is an analgesic that usually causes less stomach irritation than aspirin. Thus, it is often preferred for people with gastric ulcers or with a past history of such problems. Its antifever effect appears to be nearly as good as that of aspirin, but its anti-inflammatory effect is less strong.

As Bayer pointed out in its ads, acetaminophen has toxic effects of its own. It is not the "safe" drug that it is sometimes advertised to be. In particular, it can cause serious liver damage. Even usual doses of this drug may sometimes injure the liver. Anybody with an active liver disorder or with a liver still recovering from the long-lasting effects of liver disease should consult a doctor before taking any acetaminophen product. When taken in large overdosage by children or adults, acetaminophen has caused acute liver cell destruction, sometimes resulting in fatality.

Codeine, as we have seen, is a relatively mild narcotic. However, this drug and many of its chemical relatives, such as oxycodone, can be seriously habit forming when taken over a long period of time. Even though codeine preparations are classified as mild, these drugs present all the dependency hazards of the strong narcotic analgesics. Codeine and related drugs can create a morphine-type addiction. This hazard becomes even greater when, as often happens, these narcotics are prescribed in conjunction with a barbiturate or tranquilizer. The mind-dulling effects can be additive, and so can the dangers of dependency.

It is not uncommon for street addicts to turn to codeine or codeine-barbiturate combinations when supplies of the more usual street drugs are cut off. As with the strong narcotic pain relievers, doctors are reluctant to prescribe codeine to any patient with a history of drug abuse.

Propoxyphene (Darvon) has also been known to be involved in morphine-type dependency. This is not especially uncommon because of the extremely wide use of the drug. The most common of Darvon's unwanted side effects are dizziness, drowsiness, nausea and vomiting—all especially troublesome to the ambulatory patient. Somewhat less common are constipation, stomachache, headache, rash, visual disturbances, general weakness, fatigue, and bewildering changes in mood. Long-term intake of large doses of Darvon has been reported to cause convulsions and psychosis.

Serious overdoses of Darvon can lead, ultimately, to death. An overdose may cause stupor or coma, respiratory depression, apnea (cessation of breathing), acute circulatory failure, convulsions, irregular heartbeat, cardiac arrest, or pulmonary edema (in which the lungs fill with fluid and the patient, in effect, "drowns").

Phenacetin is sometimes used in preference to aspirin because it appears to be somewhat less toxic, and because it does not counteract the effects of gout medicines. However, it has unwanted effects of its own. After prolonged use, it may be a factor in hemolytic anemia. It has also been implicated in certain kinds of kidney damage.

Dipyrone, as I mentioned earlier, is not used routinely because of its possibly severe side effects. Among these are agranulocytosis, aplastic anemia, and thrombocytopenic purpura. Those are all serious blood disorders.

It is not necessary to continue listing all the mild analgesics and all their unwanted effects. These few examples should be enough to illustrate my point: that virtually no drug is 100 percent safe. The pain relief and muscle-spasm relief that you get from an analgesic may be welcome, but you always pay for them in one way or another. If a drug does not exhibit one side effect, it will almost certainly exhibit another. This is a major frustration of the backache drug formulary. The perfect chemical analgesic has yet to be discovered.

3. DRUGS PRESCRIBED FOR GOUT

As we saw in the last chapter, gout is an inherited disorder resulting from an error in metabolism. The body generates too much uric acid, and deposits of urate crystals lodge in the joints—including those associated with the back. The disease can cause irreversible damage to the joints in time, and even in its earlier stages may cause severe, sometimes crippling pain.

Some drugs used against gout are specific for this disease, while others are not. The main pharmacological approaches are:

1. Drugs that terminate attacks of acute gouty arthritis, by decreasing inflammation and by other means. One commonly used agent of this type is colchicine, made from roots of the meadow saffron.

2. Drugs that decrease the body's production of uric acid. Among these is allopurinol, sold under the trade name Zyloprim.

3. Drugs which, by various means, decrease the absorption of uric acid into the bloodstream and body tissues, and increase the rate at which it is passed out

of the body in urine. Among these are probenecid, sold under the trade name Benemid; and sulfinpyrazone, trade-named Anturan.

4. Drugs which, while not specific for gout, help decrease inflammation during acute attacks. None of these drugs is as effective as colchicine, but they can be useful in cases where that drug cannot be administered safely. Among these are phenylbutazone (trade names Azolid, Butazolidin) and oxyphenbutazone (Oxalid, Tandearil). These are not only good anti-inflammatory agents but are also mild analgesics. However, because they are quite toxic, they can be used only on a short-term basis.

5. General analgesics of the type we looked at in earlier sections. Both strong and mild analgesics are used in cases of gout, but there is one exception. Salicylates (aspirin and its chemical relatives) are almost never used because they tend to counteract the effects of anti-uric-acid drugs.

Side Effects and Hazards

Since many gout medicines are toxic, physicians are wary of prescribing them for pregnant women. Too little is known about their effects on an unborn baby. Fortunately, it is fairly unusual to find a woman of childbearing age suffering from gout. The disease more often attacks older people. Even when it does manifest itself at an early age, it may remain mild and uncomplicated for many years.

As I emphasized earlier, I do not advocate the abolition of all drugs, not even of strong, toxic drugs. Often they are necessary—and gout therapy is a case in point. What I do advocate is that you take no more drugs than are necessary. If you have gout, you may need regularly or frequently to take some of the drugs I have mentioned here. Your body is unavoidably being flooded with chemicals that could be doing serious damage. In this situation, it would clearly be to your advantage to avoid taking additional drugs. Instead of taking analgesic drugs to relieve pain, you could ask your doctor about using auto-acupressure as a partial or total substitute.

Though the gout medicines differ in chemical structure and in their actions in the body, their side effects tend to be similar. Gastrointestinal disturbances of various kinds are common with nearly all of these powerful drugs. Diarrhea is particularly common with colchicine in regular oral doses. This and other gout medicines also cause nausea and vomiting in many patients. They can produce or aggravate peptic ulcers. Rash is another common side effect. There may also be allergic reactions, sometimes serious ones, involving the kidneys, liver, bone marrow, cardiovascular system, and central nervous system.

4. DRUGS PRESCRIBED FOR PAGET'S DISEASE

There are two principal medications used for symptomatic treatment of Paget's disease. One is salmon calcitonin (Calcimar); the other is etidronate disodium (Didronel). Unfortunately, high doses of etidronate can cause increased pain and fractures. However, it can be given by mouth whereas calcitonin can only be administered by injection. Etidronate appears to cause fewer problems from allergic reactions and is less costly. However, the relative effectiveness of these two drugs has not yet been validated.

5. DRUGS PRESCRIBED FOR RHEUMATIC AND ARTHRITIC DISEASES

These drugs have three main purposes: (1) to reduce pain, (2) to maintain mobility in the affected joints, and (3) to prevent deformity of the joints.

As we saw in the previous chapter, the terms *rheumatic* and *arthritic* refer to a large group of disorders. The underlying causes of some of these disorders are known, enabling a physician to treat those causes. However, in other disorders, the causes are only dimly understood or are simply not known at all. In such cases, a doctor may not be able to do more than treat symptoms such as pain, stiffness, and inflammation. Or he may prescribe a drug that is thought to attack the cause of the disorder, but whose precise mechanism of action is not understood. Many anti-rheumatic-arthritic drugs are like that. We know from observation that they produce certain effects in the body, but we do not know exactly how they work.

Here are the main classes of antirheumatic and antiarthritic drugs:

A. Nonsteroidal anti-inflammatory drugs—for example, aspirin.

B. New antiarthritics of various kinds, such as:

fenoprofen (trade-named Nalfon)
ibuprofen (Motrin)
naproxen (Naprosyn)
tolmetin sodium (Tolectin)
sulindac (Clinoril)

C. Other anti-inflammatory agents such as:

phenylbutazone (Azolid, Butazoladin)
oxyphenbutazone (Oxalid, Tandearil)
indomethacin (Indocin)

D. Various anti-inflammatory drugs of unknown mechanisms of action. Prominent among these are:

penicillamine and the following gold salts:
aurothioglucose (Solganol)
gold sodium thiomalate (Myochrysine)

E. A group of drugs that are also used against malaria. Included among these are:

chloroquine (Aralan)
hydroxychloroquine (Plaquenil)

F. Certain experimental drugs that are still under investigation; for example, drugs that depress the body's immune system, which is thought to play a role in certain arthritic diseases. Among these drugs are:

cyclophosphamide (Cytoxan)
chlorambucil (Leukeran)
azathioprine (Imuran)

G. Adrenal corticosteroids. These are sometimes administered systemically; they are given by oral tablet or by injection into the muscle or bloodstream. Sometimes these medicines are given intra-articularly (injected directly into a specific joint that is giving trouble). The most commonly used systemic corticosteroids are probably prednisone and prednisolone. Some names of frequently prescribed steroids are:

betamethasone (Celestone)
cortisone (Cortone)
dexamethasone (Decadron, Dexameth)
hydrocortisone (Cortef)
methylprednisolone (Medrol)
prednisolone (Delta-Cortef)
triamcinolone (Aristocort, Kenacort)

Side Effects and Hazards

The drugs listed above are used in various ways and in many combinations. These drugs are often used in combination with aspirin or its chemical relatives. They are used for a wide variety of rheumatic, arthritic, and other disorders. These include osteoarthritis, psoriatic arthritis, juvenile rheumatoid arthritis, and ankylosing spondylitis.

The American Rheumatism Association classifies rheumatoid arthritis into four pathologic states. The severity of each stage of rheumatoid disease dictates the appropriate course of medication. Drug therapy, at the entering level or stage 1, ordinarily consists of salicylate, i.e., aspirin. At this stage, aspirin is usually given at maximum tolerated doses. This is done unless allergy, peptic ulcers, or bleeding tendencies prevent its use.

If and when the disease has progressed to a moderately severe state, stage 2, there are multiple joints involved. At that time, the more hazardous, nonsteroidal anti-inflammatory drugs discussed here may be employed. These include: phenylbutazone, oxyphenbutazone, indomethacin, and the newer nonsteroidal anti-inflammatories, such as: fenoprofen, ibuprofen, naproxen, tolmetin sodium, and sulindac. The possibility of serious toxicities must then be considered. Even potentially fatal complications, such as a total loss of production of all blood cells, must be kept in mind. Long-term therapy with the antimalarial drugs, such as chloroquine, may also be useful at this stage, although the incidence of side effects is high. At this time also, the use of intra-articular steroids (steroids injected directly into a joint space) may be considered.

As the severity of the disease progresses to stage 3, all corticosteroids or intramuscular gold therapy may be indicated. Gold compounds may be the only presently available agents that can alter or even stop the progression of this disease. Toxicity in kidney and in the bone-marrow blood-cell production centers is the limiting factor in their more widespread use.

In stage 4 of this disease, hospitalization may be recommended for administration of new investigational treatments. These include orthopedic procedures and medications such as chelating agents and immunosuppressive drugs. Examples of such drugs would be penicillamine and cyclophosphamide. Obviously, immunosuppressive drugs should only be used when more conventional treatments fail and when rapid progress of rheumatory disease results in life-threatening complications.

None of the medications we have discussed appear to reverse or even inhibit the underlying chronic and progressive inflammatory process of the rheumatic disease. Nor is the simultaneous overgrowth of tissue lining the joints and degeneration of the connective tissue of afflicted joints decreased. Drugs with the ability to fundamentally alter the degenerative destructive disease process have yet to be developed.

Many of the prescription drugs used against arthritic diseases have peculiar toxic side effects. When taken for a long period of time, some antimalarial medicines can cause damage to the retina. The damage is irreversible and can lead ultimately to blindness. These drugs act very slowly, and are not readily passed out of the body. The insidious chemical events leading to this damage can continue long after a patient has stopped taking the drug.

The antimalarial drugs can also cause gastrointestinal disturbances, headache, emotional changes and upsets, and skin rash. For this latter reason, they sometimes present problems when used against psoriatic arthritis. They may make the psoriatic skin condition worse.

Adverse reactions to penicillamine include varying degrees of allergic reactions that may be life-threatening. Skin changes may occur later in therapy with discoloration, blistering, and wrinkling. Recently, a fatal case of liver failure was reported in one patient taking penicillamine.

The gold compounds can also cause skin problems —sometimes severe ones, including complete shedding of the skin. They may also bring on various disturbances in the kidneys. Because of their toxicity and because their action in the body is not fully understood, they are seldom prescribed for children under twelve. They are rarely used for pregnant women.

The corticosteroids are another group that must be handled with extreme caution. When injected into the joints, they may bring welcome relief from pain and stiffness. However, some researchers have found that these drugs can do permanent damage to a joint if used for too long a time. Their use in this way is controversial.

Even when administered systemically (that is, with a tablet taken by mouth), these powerful steroid medicines have a number of unwanted side effects. For example, they tend to worsen hypertension (high blood pressure) and must be very carefully regulated in patients with this problem. Loss of calcium in the bones may cause spontaneous fractures. Patients with gastric or intestinal ulcers are also in potential danger from steroids. Steroids may tend to inhibit healing of ulcers in some and cause stomach ulcers in others. Diabetics must be monitored with care if given steroid therapy. The drugs oppose the effects of certain antidiabetic medicines.

Among other effects of steroids are emotional disturbances, menstrual irregularities, and (infrequently) eye cataracts after long-term use. The drugs may also bring about unwanted changes in a patient's appearance. Obesity is one possible problem. Another is hirsutism, which is the abnormal growth of hair on the face and other parts of the body. Still other side effects of steroids are a moon-faced appearance, and a "buffalo hump" at the back of the neck. Those effects are caused by redistribution of body fat and fluids.

The side effects of all drugs are particularly hazardous in children. Juvenile rheumatoid arthritis is a serious disease requiring strong medication. Once again, I emphasize that such medication may be necessary despite the unwanted effects. Still, anything that can be done to reduce the total load of drugs in the body is welcome. Among the special dangers of antirheumatic drugs in children are the following: gastric hemorrhage, liver damage, disturbances of growth and endocrine balance, loss of calcium in the bones, and decreased resistance to infection.

The antimalarial drug, chloroquine, can be fatal in overdosage, and children are especially sensitive to it. Thus, any adult taking this medicine at home should be especially careful to keep it out of children's reach.

The elderly are also susceptible to the side effects of many rheumatic-arthritic medications. This is unfortunate, for these diseases often grow progressively worse with age. This is the paradox with which a physician and an elderly patient must too often wrestle: when you are old and need drug treatment the most, you are least able to tolerate that treatment.

DRUGS

Alka-Seltzer, 83
Amid-Sal, 80
Anacin, 79
Anturan, 88
A.P.C., 81
Aralan, 91
Aristocort, 91
Arthritis Strength Bufferin, 79
A.S.A., 79, 82
Ascodeen-30, 82
Ascriptin, 83
Ascriptin with codeine, 82
Aspirin Free Anacin 3, 80
Azolid, 88, 90
Benemid, 88
Bufferin, 79, 83
Butazolidin, 88, 90
Calcimar, 89
Celestone, 91
Clinoril, 90
Cope, 79

Cortef, 91
Cortone, 91
Cytoxan, 91
Darvocet-N, 82
Darvon, 78, 86
Darvon with A.S.A., 82
Darvon Compound, 82
Darvon-N, 78
Darvon-N with A.S.A., 82
Datril, 80, 85
Decadron, 91
Delta-Cortef, 91
Dem-A.P.A.P., 81
Demerol, 75, 81
Dexameth, 91
Didronel, 89
Dilaudid, 75
Dolene, 78
Dolene Compound 65, 82
Dolophine, 75, 78
Ecotrin, 79

CHAPTER 9

Brief Comments on Nonprescription Drugs, Gadgets, and Other Home Remedies

The amounts of pills, liniments, body trusses, exercise gadgets and other backache "cures" sold in this country are so enormous that it is virtually impossible to total them. Estimates of the dollar value vary widely. One respected medical encyclopedia guesses that Americans afflicted with arthritis (and those who believe they are so afflicted) spend some $250 million a year on *misrepresented* products alone. The amount spent on legitimate products is probably at least that large or larger. Another estimate is that, in any one year, at least one adult in three buys *something* for back pain. The "something" may be a 98-cent bottle of aspirin or a 600-dollar orthopedic bed or thousands of dollars' worth of professional medical treatment and drugs.

The difficulty in arriving at a reliable estimate arises partly from the fact that not all the products are sold exclusively for back pains. Aspirin has many uses, of course. Arthritis remedies attract people with aches and pains in any part of the body.

Let us look at some of these products and their hazards.

Analgesics are sold in enormous quantities in the United States—and, for that matter, also in Europe, Russia, Japan, and Australia. The most popular non-prescription analgesic is aspirin. As we discussed in Chapter 8, in the United States there are approximately 50,000 over-the-counter medications in which aspirin is a primary agent. The second most popular nonprescription analgesic is acetaminophen, sold under the trade names Tylenol and Datril. In the last chapter, we studied the unwanted side effects of these analgesics. Many people assume that these drugs would not be widely advertised and sold if they were unsafe. As we have seen, these assumptions are not warranted.

At a recent annual meeting of the Arthritis Foundation, a noted expert in gastroenterology warned a large gathering of rheumatologists about severe damage to the stomach lining that may result from aspirin usage. His studies included direct inspection of the stomach lining with a gastroscope. He found severe damage occurred in some arthritic patients who took aspirin and other nonsteroidal, anti-inflammatory drugs for as few as 7 days. Aspirin caused the most extensive irritation, scoring 58.5 out of a possible maximum score of 60 points.

One of the most important findings of that study was that patients' subjective complaints did not always correspond with the findings of injury on direct inspection of the stomach lining. Some subjects who had severe damage to the stomach reported little or no discomfort. It was thought that these findings may explain how gastric bleeding and sudden stomach perforation may occur without the patient's prior awareness of a serious problem.

If you have not read the discussion of nonprescription drugs in Chapter 8, you may not be aware of how aspirin and acetaminophen have contributed to so many fatalities. You may find pages 83–85 especially informative. I strongly urge you to review the scope and severity of these hazards.

Vitamin preparations are best sellers in the nonprescription drug market. Very large doses of vitamins have been promoted for use in people who do *not* have vitamin deficiencies. The use of vitamins in huge doses is often referred to as megavitamin therapy. A vitamin megadose may be defined as one which is ten or more times the recommended daily allowance. Most people do not appreciate that megavitamin therapy can be quite dangerous. Many physicians consider vitamin toxicity a widespread problem and routinely quiz all patients about vitamin intake.

The Recommended Daily Allowance (RDA) for Vitamin A is 1,400 to 5,000 International Units (IU). There are tablets on the market containing up to 50,000 IU. Some manufacturers recommend megadosage up to 400,000 units.

An excessive intake of Vitamin A can lead to a poisoning disorder known as Hypervitaminosis A. This disorder was first identified in 1944. Reported cases in children were associated with Vitamin A intakes of 50,000 to 500,000 units per day.

In children, excessive Vitamin A intake can lead to increased pressure inside the head with resultant headaches and swelling of the optic nerve. In infants, Vitamin A toxicity can cause lethargy and coma.

In adults, the symptoms of toxicity from Vitamin A may be fatigue, headache, and loss of appetite. There may be skin problems including dryness and discoloration. Hypervitaminosis A may also be associated with bone and joint pains and increased destruction of bone. Furthermore, chronic liver disease leading to cirrhosis has been reported. Cirrhosis of the liver is a chronic disease characterized by the destruction of normal liver tissue and the development of abnormal scarring.

The RDA for Vitamin D is 400 units daily. Some tablets come in a 50,000-unit size. Many medical authorities feel that even Vitamin D enriched foods may cause problems.

The continued daily ingestion of Vitamin D in a dose of 150,000 units or more may result in poisoning. The long-term administration of excessive quantities of Vitamin D leads to a serious disorder of calcium metabolism. It is called Hypervitaminosis D.

The early symptoms of Hypervitaminosis D may be headache, fatigue, weakness, nausea, vomiting, and diarrhea. Later, kidney function is progressively impaired. There may be calcium deposits formed in soft tissues. This frequently leads to the formation of kidney stones. Other sites of calcification may include blood vessels, heart muscle, lungs and skin. In 23 percent of patients, there is a generalized osteoporosis (loss of minerals from bones). There is a localized osteoporosis in an additional 41 percent of Hypervitaminosis D cases.

The RDA for Vitamin C is 35 to 45 milligrams (mg.). It is available in tablets of 50 to 1,000 mg. Some manufacturers recommend the routine use of 3,000 mg. daily. They suggest taking 6,000 mg. a day during a respiratory infection.

According to physicians, Vitamin C toxicity can lead to kidney stones and destruction of the antianemia vitamin, B_{12}. Some people complain of gastric (stomach) upset and also of urinary bladder irritation. Megadoses of Vitamin C may enhance fertility by thinning the mucus of the womb, and are alleged to trigger diabetes mellitus (sugar diabetes). Excessive intake of Vitamin C can produce false results in laboratory tests of blood, urine, and stool.

The RDA for Vitamin E is 400 units. Tablets come in 50 to 1,000 units. Manufacturers recommend up to 1,000 units daily. Symptoms of Vitamin E overdosage are said to include nausea, blurred vision, fatigue and slower blood clotting.

Niacin is a member of the Vitamin B complex. It is also known as nicotinic acid. The RDA for niacin is 5 to 20 mg. Tablets are available in 100 to 500 mg. sizes. Some manufacturers recommend up to 2,000 mg. per day. The effects of niacin overdosage include flushing, itching, nausea, heartburn and diarrhea. Other toxic effects are reported to be abnormal blood sugar tolerance and liver damage.

Liniments, such as Ben-Gay, Minit-Rub, Musterole and Heet, are popular with back pain sufferers. The major active ingredient of most such products is methylsalicylate. This chemical causes a temporary, usually harmless, irritation in the skin, making small blood vessels dilate and giving a pleasant sensation of heat. Whether the heat itself has any effect on painful joints or deep-lying muscles is not a matter of universal agreement. Possibly the physical massage with which a liniment is applied does as much good as the liniment itself. But many people do report that they get mild, temporary, beneficial effects from over-the-counter liniments.

Like almost all drugs, however, the popular rub-ons have unwanted properties and some are dangerous. These chemicals are decidedly poisonous if swallowed. The skin irritant, methylsalicylate, will cause painful and possible dangerous burns if it gets on mucous membranes, such as those of the mouth and nose. These potential hazards are excellent reasons for keeping these drugs far away from children. Most people can put liniments on the skin of their backs and limbs without damage. However, some will find that an unpleasant itching or burning rash will appear. Sometimes this occurs after one application; sometimes it develops after repeated use over a span of days. The rash signals, of course, that the chemical is doing damage and that its use should be discontinued immediately. No such liniment should be applied over cuts or scratches or on skin that is irritated from some other cause.

Liniments containing both methylsalicylate and local skin anesthetic agents are also sold for "arthritis relief." A familiar example is the commercial preparation known as Exocaine. It contains benzocaine. The use of "caine" rub-on anesthetics tends to sensitize people to these drugs. Once an allergy is developed, further use is generally best avoided. Because of this, some people cannot have medical or dental anesthesia with drugs such as novocaine and xylocaine.

Devices, gadgets and gimmicks range from the demonstrably useful to the ridiculous, the questionable, and the downright fraudulent.

Many backache sufferers say they have been helped by orthopedic mattresses, chairs that are designed to improve the sitting posture, and posture-improving shoes. Others say they have benefited by taking certain courses of exercises, massages, or chiropractic manipulations. Still others have reached for more mystical cures. Among products on the market is a copper bracelet that is said to relieve arthritis. There is also a pyramid-shaped arrangement of wire that purportedly will cure various ills, including backache, if you lie within it.

Some of these products and services have a valid scientific rationale to recommend them; others offer a rationale that sounds sensible, but turns out to be nonsense on closer examination. Still others offer nothing but hope. My advice is that you consult your doctor before spending money on any such product or service.

If you buy indiscriminately, you could not only lose money but also make your back problems worse. An awkwardly shaped chair, touted as "orthopedic" or "doctor-recommended for posture," might in fact aggravate certain back disorders. Serious injuries may result from an inept massage or an inexpertly designed set of exercises.

In the next three chapters, we will return to the examination of physician-prescribed treatments. We will consider some procedures offered by anesthesiologists, orthopedic surgeons, and neurosurgeons.

CHAPTER **10**

Nonsurgical Procedures for Relief of Back Pains: Spinal Injections of Medication

Nonsurgical procedures for the relief of back pains were developed by physicians as a response to disappointment with the therapeutic results of surgery. Two logical approaches to the problems of nonsurgical therapy have been employed. The first attempts to remove the cause; and the second strives to modify the response to that cause.

A significant attempt at the first approach was the development of the procedure called chemonucleolysis. It was initially reported on by Dr. L. Smith in 1963. In that procedure, chymopapain—an enzyme which converts proteins into smaller molecules—was injected through the skin directly into an involved herniated disc. The chymopapain injection often successfully liquefied the substance of the herniated nucleus pulposus (the central portion of the disc). The result was a chemical (nonsurgical) method of relieving the compression of the affected spinal cord or nerve roots. Dr. Smith reported complete relief in 83 percent of his patients. Many investigators were not able to duplicate his results.

Chymopapain has significant potential hazards. Consequently, it is not currently available for medical use in the United States. One major difficulty is the destructive effect chymopapain has on blood vessels. Some researchers discovered a correlation between the concentration of chymopapain and damage to small blood vessels. Others reported findings ranging from minute capillary bleeding and microthrombi (small clots located in capillaries) to significant hemorrhage.

Medical specialists documented that the chemonucleolysis procedure was usually extremely painful and required the administration of a general anesthetic. Severe temporary exacerbation of pain was common. In most patients, for the first 12 to 36 hours after injection, there was a significant incidence of severe lumbar muscular spasm. There were also rare complications including disc space infection and injury to the spinal cord and spinal nerves. Most unfortunately, however, there was a 1 to 2 percent rate of anaphylaxis, a life-threatening allergic reaction associated with the chemonucleolysis.

The second approach to nonsurgical therapy treats the inflammation of the spinal nerve root, rather than the primary cause of that inflammation. Anesthesiologists have developed procedures of injecting medications. Procaine is used to produce nerve blocks, and steroids are used to reduce inflammation. Currently, these types of injections are widely used in pain clinics.

Pain relief from sciatica is sought by injection of steroids into coverings of and around the spinal canal and nerve roots. Whether the injection should be epidural or intrathecal (in the subarachnoid space) will be decided upon by complicated diagnostic procedures. Epidural injections are given outside of the dura—the outermost of the three membranes covering the spinal cord. Injections in the subarachnoid space are placed between the arachnoid—the second of the three membranes covering the spinal cord—and the innermost spinal membrane.

The degree of relief obtained from spinal injections naturally varies from patient to patient. In some studies, there were significant differences in how many injections were required to obtain pain relief. The site of injections, the technique of injections, and the medications injected are all important considerations.

Unquestionably, these techniques of intradural and extradural injection of steroids may have something significant to offer the patient seeking pain relief from sciatica. Patients with sciatica are urged to consult their physicians as to whether the injection of steroids around the spinal cord or spinal roots would be appropriate for their particular problems.

However, these techniques are not without their hazards. One significant hazard is the development of infection around the site of injection. A severe infection leading to epidural abscess runs a dramatic course of high fever, chills, and an onset of paralysis. According to some experts, the development of a low grade infection is more common. Infection may be introduced into the epidural space during blocking techniques. If such low grade infection takes place, often regardless of the site of injection, the following is a typical course of illness: from 5 to 10 days after the injection, the patient will notice an increase in pain with radiation into both arms or both legs, depending upon the site of injection. Usually, the patient does not have chills or fever and does not develop paralysis. If, however, the exacerbation of the pain continues, it will require epidural (spinal) taps to obtain specimens of the infecting organism. Ordinarily, long-term antibiotic therapy to control or help abolish the infection will be utilized.

CHAPTER 11

Surgical Procedures for Relief of Back Pains: Diskectomies, Laminectomies, and Spinal Fusions

Operations may be necessary to alleviate such diverse conditions as spondylolisthesis, spinal fractures, arthritic deformities, tumors, and vascular obstructions. Operations for relief of back pains are as varied as the underlying causes. Surgery for pain relief is ordinarily done only when there is a failure of conservative (that is, medical) therapy. An urgent need for operative treatment may arise when there is significant muscle paralysis. A most common surgery performed for relief of back pains is the removal of a herniated disc.

Rupture of intervertebral discs can occur in the cervical and thoracic spine, but are most common in the lumbar spine. They occur between the bodies of the fourth and fifth lumbar vertebrae, and the bodies of the fifth lumbar vertebra and the sacrum. We discussed the structure of our backs in Chapter 4, and the mechanisms of disc damage in Chapter 5.

A diskectomy includes the removal of both the extruded nucleus pulposus and the interior contents of the affected disc. Surgical dissection of the back may require the removal of bone, if it is impossible to approach the disc through the space between vertebral laminas. The excision of the posterior arch of a vertebra is called a laminectomy. If the herniated disc protrudes in the midline, bilateral (two-sided) exposure is usually necessary for complete removal.

A spinal fusion may be done at the same time as a diskectomy. Usually, it is done with bone grafts that are removed from the ilium (hip bone). Following a simple diskectomy, a patient is usually allowed to walk within a few days. After a spinal fusion, many orthopedic surgeons prescribe several weeks at bed rest, and apply a brace or cast before allowing ambulation.

Removal of a herniated disc, with or without spinal fusion, does not guarantee freedom from back pains. Many studies have found that approximately 40 percent of patients did *not* regard themselves as "cured" by operation. Moreover, 5 to 10 percent of patients reported that their pain was either unchanged or intensified after surgery. Some patients complain of increasing discomfort despite multiple laminectomies. The worst results are often found in cases where financial compensation for injuries is directly involved. About 70 percent of such patients fail to achieve complete recovery with surgery.

When the original symptoms persist immediately after a diskectomy and when they fail to subside, surgeons consider several possibilities. There may have been a failure to remove the offending disc. There may have been a second herniated disc or an unrecognized tumor that was not removed. There may have been surgical trauma to the nerve root at the time of the operation.

Long-term recovery after diskectomy is difficult to assess because some symptoms are relieved at the time of surgery, only to recur after a variable period. Physical causes for recurrent symptoms include insufficient removal of disc contents with further herniation. Others are rupture of another disc, adhesions about the nerve root and osteophyte (bone spur) formation at the laminectomy site.

If surgery is necessary for recurrent symptoms after a diskectomy, the second operation is usually more extensive. If a previous spinal fusion was performed, the resultant bony mass must be removed. The spinal cord requires extensive exploration. That involves a meticulous excision of scar tissue, and freeing of the nerve tissue above the previously operated area. Frequently, there is an excision of the lamina of the first normal vertebra above the original site. If extensive removal of the posterior vertebral arches is necessary, complex spinal fusions may be done with bone grafts from the sacrum.

Following surgery, the patient may need to be immobilized in a spica cast extending from the nipple line to the knee on one side. Straight leg-raising exercises of the opposite leg are utilized to minimize the possibility of postoperative adhesions forming around the nerve roots.

Sometimes, a spinal fusion is postponed until the results of the first part of the surgery can be evaluated. If there is a need for further stabilization, another operation is performed. At that time, fusion between the vertebral bodies may be utilized.

Following all diskectomies, patients are advised to regard their backs with care. Generally, patients are advised to avoid all lifting in a stooped position, all heavy pushing and shoveling for at least 9 months. The recommendations given in Chapter 25, "Living with Our Vulnerable Backs," would be well taken.

In this chapter, we discussed surgical operations that remove causes of back pains. In the next chapter, we will briefly examine the currently available neurosurgical procedures for interrupting pain pathways.

CHAPTER **12**

Neurosurgical Procedures for Relief of Back Pains: Interrupting Pain Pathways

There are a number of currently available neurosurgical procedures for interrupting pain pathways. They are essentially destructive procedures because parts of the nervous system are permanently destroyed. This destruction may produce various consequences which are unwanted. If there are any mistakes, the wrong pathways may be interrupted. There may be losses of muscle control, of muscle strength, and of sensation. Psychosurgery (surgery of the brain) is perhaps the most drastic of the neurosurgical operations for pain relief. These are very drastic procedures which may alter personality as well as pain.

There are a number of techniques that have been utilized to relieve chronic and intractable pain disorders. Leukotomy is the cutting of nerve fibers crossing from one hemisphere of the brain to the other. Stereotactic cingulumotomy is the precise positioning of nerve pathway destruction in the sensation-carrying area of the brain called the cingulum. Leukotomy and stereotactic cingulumotomy are two of the more commonly used psychosurgical techniques. After such surgery, pain is still perceived. However, the person no longer interprets the pain as suffering.

A neurosurgical relief of pain can also be obtained from those operations which sever pain tracts in the spinal cord. Anterolateral cordotomy is a surgical procedure that abolishes both pain and temperature sensations. Generally, it is carried out at the level of the neck. This technique can be done by a newer and less traumatic procedure using radio frequencies to perform a surgical destruction. It has been reported that in well-selected cases, this procedure can bring immediate relief of pain to 85 percent of people. However, there is a 35–40 percent recurrence rate within 6 months. Cutting both sides of the cord in the high neck region must be avoided since it may cause severe respiratory failure and a consequent inability of the person to sustain life.

Commissural myelotomy is another procedure for relieving pain by cutting into the spinal cord. In the technique, a specific part of the cord is sectioned. Spinothalamic fibers are cut as they cross within the spinal cord from the nerve root (dorsal horn) to the spinothalamic tract. It requires a midline exact-center incision of the spinal cord. In situations where the fibers are not totally destroyed surgically and part of the pathway is left intact, this technique carries a significant risk of aggravating the pain problem. As previously mentioned, inadvertent destruction of motor nerve fibers may cause paralysis.

Dorsal rhizotomy is the cutting of spinal nerve roots containing sensory fibers. It is a surgical procedure that is often utilized in relieving pain arising from isolated but severely injured nerve roots. In most studies, the long-term success rate does not exceed 30 percent, even though early relief of pain has been achieved in as many as 65 percent of patients. Because there is overlapping of the segmental innervation from one spinal root to another, at least three adjacent roots of spinal nerves must be sectioned. Therefore, this technique usually requires the removal of the spinal lamina at four or more levels of vertebrae. Obviously, this is a very major neurosurgical procedure, and such extensive surgery may be fraught with complications.

CHAPTER **13**

Pain Relief with Electrostimulation: Living Better Electrically

One of the space-age spin-offs related to acupuncture therapy is the use of electric stimulation to decrease pain. For centuries, the potent analgesic effect resulting from peripheral nerve stimulation has been produced with inserted acupuncture needles. It was not until the late 1960s that the technique of applying electric current to peripheral nerves directly through the skin was utilized for pain relief. Presently, electric stimulation is delivered by a machine called a transcutaneous electric neurostimulator, abbreviated as TENS.

Low-intensity stimulation, applied for long periods, selectively activates large nerve fibers. According to current theories of Ronald Melzack and Patrick Wall, such nerve stimulation closes the mechanism called the "pain gate" in the spinal cord. High-intensity stimulation is usually applied for short periods only. It stimulates the brain predominantly through small nerve fibers. Though this procedure may be somewhat painful in itself, it usually triggers inhibitory transmission of more powerful pain stimuli arising from other areas. Most probably, both these types of stimulation also release endorphins, the naturally occurring pain-relieving substances which are manufactured in the brain.

We have already mentioned that physicians have a great deal of experience in trying to reduce or eliminate pain by doing surgical procedures directly on the cord or nerve roots that deal with sensation. Because motor nerve fibers run parallel to the sensory ones in the spinal cord, surgery runs real risks of producing muscular weakness and even paralysis. If motor roots serving the muscles are severed, muscular weakness and/or paralysis may result. Even with successful operations, the pain-relieving effects of surgery directly on the spinal cord frequently wear off after a period of time, such as 6 months to a year. Consequently, operations are usually reserved for special pain situations, such as those associated with cancer or with tic douloureux.

The use of electrostimulators has been incorporated in a number of newer surgical procedures. In one surgical procedure, the electrodes are placed inside the brain in an area that controls the brain's appreciation of pain. These operations sometimes result in favorable effects. Oftentimes, a patient can activate the electrostimulator and reduce or eliminate his awareness of pain for a time. Unfortunately, some patients have found that after periods of relative freedom from pain, they could no longer tolerate the implanted electrodes. Some patients have complained that such operations have made them feel peculiar and not in control. This may be related to an excessive production of pain-relieving substances, endorphins. Excessive endorphins might possibly resemble being on an opiate high. Other patients reported that although they got initial relief from their implanted stimulator within the brain, the pain returned after a variable period of time. Some patients observed that their pain was even worse than before the operation.

Less drastic surgery involves the implantation of fine wire electrodes directly into the spinal cord above the level of pain. These electrodes are attached to a small receiver beneath the skin of the back. A transmitter may be taped over the receiver, and the transmitter can be programmed to send electric signals into the spine when a switch is turned on. The patient can wear a control transmitter, or carry it in a pocket or a purse, or keep it on a bedside stand. Such stimulators, connected directly to the dorsal column of pain-bearing fibers within the spinal cord, are called dorsal column stimulators, and abbreviated DCS.

No surgical procedure is necessary for the use of TENS (transcutaneous electric neurostimulators) for they are merely taped to the skin. TENS may be placed over the spine or any painful area. Again, the patient has complete control as to how long to utilize the electric stimulation and how intense to make the current. Many patients enjoy partial relief some of the time. Some get complete relief some of the time. However, most people do not get complete relief *any* of the time.

Transcutaneous electric stimulation should never be used without your physician's approval. TENS should not be used by people with cardiac pacemakers, bladder stimulators, or other electronic medical devices.

Some problems my patients have encountered with the use of TENS involve skin irritation and skin burns. Such burns sometimes may result when there is inadequate preparation of the skin to allow easy current flow through the transcutaneous stimulator. What is most disturbing, however, is that patients who sometimes get relief from their pain problems can get a rebound effect. The rebound effect occurs when the electro-stimulator is shut off, and the painful condition is intensified. At times, the patient may know when the rebound effect is going to occur because the TENS loses its effectiveness in reducing pain although it is still operating.

There are special uses for the transcutaneous electric stimulator that are compatible with the auto-acupressure system of pain relief as demonstrated in this book. If a person is not able to utilize the auto-acupressure system because he is psychologically or physically unable to apply adequate pressure, electric stimulation with a TENS might be employed. I do not recommend using it on the ear system of points. Currently available electrostimulators I have seen have much too large an area of contact. They do not ordinarily apply the specific kinds of stimulation needed for ear areas. They might produce skin burns in areas of decreased electrical resistance, such as the appropriate auto-acupressure stimulation points. I do not think it is a good idea to use large amounts of electric current on the external ear since I do not know how it might affect mechanisms of the internal ear. Theoretically, large TENS output applied to the skull could affect brain mechanisms directly, but this is not very probable. Nevertheless, it is not a clinical experiment I would recommend being performed. Moreover, I have observed that excessive electrostimulation on ear system points produced rebound effects.

The use of electrostimulation on the auto-acupressure body system of points might well be appropriate for those people who are unable to do auto-acupressure techniques. I have seen patients who, because of arthritic conditions of the hands, advanced age, or infirmity, were unable to apply adequate stimulation for auto-acupressure. If you are unable to perform auto-acupressure techniques, you should request your physician's advice as to an appropriate TENS for your personal use. Your physician may recommend one of the newly designed advanced electronic solid-state TENS that are small and are able to be hand held. Such stimulators have the advantage of being portable and thereby being available for use in many situations. For example, someone who develops low back pain while riding in a car on a highway might relieve the pain quite promptly with the administration of electrostimulation to an auto-acupressure body point, such as *Knee 1* or *Thigh 1*.

It should be remembered, however, that although I have not seen the problem of the rebound effect from the use of auto-acupressure, I have seen this effect from the use of electrostimulation. It is strongly urged that periods of electrostimulation of auto-acupressure points be short, rather than long. It must be emphasized again that people with cardiac pacemakers, bladder stimulators, or other medical electronic devices should *not* use transcutaneous electric stimulation.

We have already mentioned obtaining pain relief with the use of the auto-acupressure systems of ear points and body points. In Chapter 3, you learned why auto-acupressure relieves back pains. Now it is time to learn how to utilize these systems. We will first discuss basic principles of relieving back pains with auto-acupressure. Then we will detail the methods of location and self-stimulation of the various points.

CHAPTER **14**

The Basic Principles of Relieving Back Pains with Auto-Acupressure

You are now about to learn a new way of relieving back pains. Since it is new to you, you should expect an initial period of unfamiliarity and awkwardness. During this period, your results may be disappointing.

This initial period is, in effect, a period of "apprenticeship." It is quite brief for most people. But I want to be very sure you are prepared for it. There is almost always such a period. Auto-acupressure utilizes the application of acupuncturelike techniques to oneself. It is not a particularly difficult skill to master, but it is a skill; it must be learned. Your confidence and the sureness of your fingers and thumbs will improve with practice. So will the efficacy of the technique in relieving pain and muscle spasm.

I make a point of this because I do not want you to give in to early disappointment. This is not a book of quackery. It makes no promises that it cannot fulfill. Some of my patients have used words like "miraculous" and "magical" in describing auto-acupressure, and some have talked about "instant" relief, but to promise such results would be foolhardy. Auto-acupressure depends on the proper stimulation of nerves at certain very carefully chosen body points or loci.

Except by luck, you are not likely to find the loci precisely or stimulate them in the right way the first time you try.

When you do become skilled with the technique, however, you will find that the relief may come faster and more surely than is possible with pills.

In the next chapters, you will find illustrated descriptions of the major locations to stimulate for relief of back pains, along with specific instructions dealing with stimulation of each locus. This chapter is devoted to general directions. Be sure to familiarize yourself thoroughly with what is said here before attempting your first self-treatment.

PREPARATIONS

If you are under a doctor's care for your back problem, ask his advice before you start using auto-acupressure. This is only common sense. In designing your course of treatment, he may well have had to balance many factors against each other. To make *any* change without consulting him would be foolish and might be dangerous. It is likely that your physician will endorse your use of auto-acupressure. However, he might want to make certain other changes in your treatment program to accommodate this new element. Auto-acupressure should be included as part of a total medical treatment program.

Be wary of making abrupt changes in your drug-taking regimen, especially if you are on prescription drugs. You are quite likely to find that auto-acupressure can replace analgesics and muscle relaxants. But *do not* stop taking any prescribed drug until the doctor who prescribed it has said you may. One reason for this is that abrupt withdrawal from some drugs can be physically dangerous. Another reason is that many drugs have multiple effects. While auto-acupressure can control pain and muscle spasm, it may not produce other effects that your doctor feels are needed. Your doctor may be delighted to have you reduce your daily intake of analgesics, but he may want you to take some medication to reduce inflammation.

THE THUMBNAIL TECHNIQUE

Auto-acupressure is derived from acupuncture. However, it would be very dangerous for most people to stimulate themselves with needles. Needle acupuncture should be administered only under the watchful eye of a physician. For that reason, in treating your back pains you will be using your thumbnails instead of needles.

Be sure you understand this clearly. Pressing with the fleshy pads or bony tips of your thumbs may have little or no effect on the nerves you are attempting to stimulate. You *must* use the nails.

Your thumbnails should be short and rounded so that you do not injure yourself with your own nails. To make certain you do not, I would counsel against trying this technique with long or pointed nails. Plastic nail extenders are definitely hazardous. When auto-acupressure is properly applied, there is *no* bruising, puncturing, or other injury to the skin.

Your thumbs should be *bent* when applying auto-acupressure. This is illustrated in Fig. 1.

The human hand is built in such a way that the thumb can apply maximum pressure when in this bent position. To improve the leverage still more, I will suggest various ways in which you can oppose the pressure from your thumb with answering pressure from your fingers. For example, when your bent thumb is pressing the thumbnail into a point on one side of your leg, your fingers will be wrapped around the other side.

FIGURE 1

HOW MUCH PRESSURE?

You must press on the indicated points hard enough to make them hurt briefly. As you will discover, some of them will be exquisitely tender. (In fact, the tenderness will be a signal that you have hit the given locus with precision.) Do not worry: the pain will not last long, and your reward for enduring it will be the alleviation of much longer-lasting pain in your back. But you *must* be willing to press hard enough to affect the nerve at the indicated locus. Insufficient pressure will not produce the desired effects.

HOW LONG?

Maintain hard pressure for 30 seconds at each acupressure point.

If you find it difficult to maintain pressure steadily for that long a time, try a rhythmic off–on technique instead. In this technique, you increase and decrease the pressure once a second throughout the 30-second period. Push hard; then ease off; then push again.

CHOOSING AUTO-ACUPRESSURE POINTS

In the next chapters, you will find descriptions and illustrations of pairs of points in various parts of the back, thighs, legs, and ears. Obviously, you will not want to use all of these points every time your back aches. Instead, you should choose among them on the basis of two main questions:

1. *Which are most effective for me?* An excellent way to start answering this question is to experiment. Start with those points that are the most tender when your back is aching. They are tender because they are on nerve pathways that are being stimulated by referred pain from the site of the back disorder. These particular points are most likely to produce results when stimulated by auto-acupressure.

Having found which are the most tender points, experiment with various combinations. You should be able to find two or three pairs of points that have a clear effect on your backache. If there are no points that seem clearly more tender than the others, then it will be a process of trial and error. However, most people discover highly effective points quite rapidly.

2. *Which are easiest for me to stimulate?* Not everybody is shaped alike. All people do not have the same dexterity and muscular strength in their hands. Not all points are equally accessible to all men and women. Furthermore, as a back pain sufferer, you may well have more stiffness in the back and hips on some days than on others. A point you could reach easily yesterday may seem inaccessible today.

If you discover that several different pairs of points give you approximately equal results, choose among them on the basis of accessibility. If a point seems hard for you to reach and is awkward to stimulate, abandon the point. Work with others that are more accessible.

PAIRING

I have used the phrase *pairs of points,* and now I will explain what I mean by it. With exceptions, most acupressure points come in matched pairs: one on the left side of the body and a corresponding point on the right. For example, one backache locus is behind the left knee, and the matching one is behind the right knee.

As a general rule, you will usually find points most tender on the side of the body where the back pain is. If your back pain is clearly one-sided, you might feel it sharply on the right side, perhaps radiating downward through the right buttock. In that case, you might find that all or most of the pressure points on your right side are much more tender than the matching ones on the left. If that is so, you may find that you can obtain adequate or complete relief simply by applying auto-acupressure to those right-side points. However, if the points on the opposite side are more sensitive than normal, the most complete pain relief may be obtained from stimulating both sides.

There may be a crossover effect. Your pain might be on one side, and the most tender acupressure points might be on the opposite side. For example, your pain is on the right side, but your most tender points are on the left side. When that is the case, it is possible that you may obtain relief just by stimulating the points on the left side. Again, it is much more likely that stimulation of acupressure points on both the right and left sides will obtain the best results.

It may also happen that your back pain is not clearly located on either side. It may feel centered or diffused, with no readily apparent location at all. In this case, there is not likely too much difference between left and right in the tenderness of the loci. Some pairs may be more tender than other pairs, as we noted earlier; but the two points in each pair are likely to be quite evenly matched. In any situation such as this, where there is anything less than a perfectly clear difference in tenderness from left to right, you should press *both* points in each pair.

REPEAT APPLICATIONS

When you follow the directions in this book, it is impossible to "overdose" yourself with auto-acupressure. This is not true of drugs, of course.

If you find that an initial application of auto-acupressure has not given you adequate relief (which is likely to happen frequently during your apprenticeship period, less often later), you simply repeat the process. When one application begins to "wear off," you should be able to give yourself another with perfect safety.

If an initial application has not worked well, you may find it helpful to vary the technique or loci the second time you try. This will be especially useful in your early, experimental period. If you used steady pressure the first time, try the rhythmic off–on technique the next time. If you pressed only the points on one side and did not get sufficient pain relief, stimulate the points on both sides during the repeat application.

POSITION

All of the points should be pressed while you are sitting or lying down. As we go through the points one by one, I will describe the positions that most people seem to find the most effective. You can vary these if you wish. However, do not try to apply pressure while standing.

This concludes our discussion of basic principles. You are now ready to learn how to relieve your back pains with the auto-acupressure system of body points.

CHAPTER **15**

Relieving Back Pains with the Auto-Acupressure System of Body Points: Methods of Location

The Auto-Acupressure System of Body Points deals with large nerves that become involved in back pain. One such nerve is the sciatic, whose branches and subdivisions make it by far the longest nerve pathway in the body. The auto-acupressure points in this body system are all points where branches of such nerves come close enough to the skin surface to be accessible to thumbnail pressure.

In the pages that follow, I will describe the system of body points one by one, giving you directions to help you find each point. Follow the directions as carefully as you can, referring to the drawings for further guidance. As I mentioned in the last chapter, it is *essential* that you locate each point precisely. Even a very small deviation from the target could lessen the thumbnail pressure's effects and sometimes make the entire process ineffective. In auto-acupressure, a miss is as good as a mile. For full effect, you must learn to press exactly on the points where nerves are most fully exposed.

This will not be as difficult as it sounds. Your body will tell you when you are on target. When you learn to recognize them, the signals will be virtually unmistakable.

To some degree, every auto-acupressure point is more sensitive to thumbnail pressure than are the surrounding areas. This is true even when your back is not aching and the nerves are not in a particularly irritated state. When you press your thumbnail firmly and precisely into one of the designated points, you will feel a peculiar sensation of tenderness. To many people, the sensation is something like the tingling that results when you hit the "funny bone" at the back of your elbow. That odd feeling does not come from hitting bone, but from hitting a nerve that is exposed between the bones in the elbow joint. The sensation seems to spread down the outer side of your arm, sometimes into the palm of your hand and down the little finger. The sensation that results from thumbnailing an acupressure point is seldom quite so dramatic but is similar. There is a feeling of having hit a nerve, which is precisely what you have done.

At times when your back is aching, many or most of those same points will become especially tender. Thus, if you have trouble locating any point when you are not actually suffering from back pain, wait until the next backache strikes. Then you are likely to find that some hard-to-find points are signaling their positions with great clarity.

MEASURING

It is essential in auto-acupressure (as in traditional acupuncture) to locate points *exactly*. If you are even as little as a quarter-inch off target, in many cases, you may get disappointing results.

This chapter makes use of drawings to help you find the acupressure points on your own body. I will also give written directions. In doing so, I will use certain units of measurement that may be unfamiliar to you; they may seem puzzlingly imprecise. I will be talking about *finger widths* and *finger inches*. What are they? Why do I use them instead of more familiar units?

The reason for using them is not hard to explain. Human beings do not come in one standard size. A given acupressure point might be 6 inches from the knee in somebody with long legs, but only 4 inches in somebody with short legs. Thus, any attempt to use fixed units of measurement such as inches would lead us into confusion.

Though people differ in size and shape, however, certain body *relationships* are almost always constant. Certain dimensions of the hands, for example, tend to maintain a quite constant relationship with other body dimensions in a given person. Thus, if you use your hands to measure distances on *your* body, you are likely to arrive at the same points as somebody else using his hands to mark off distances on *his* body. That occurs even though the two of you differ in stature and other dimensions.

Hence my use of variable rather than fixed units of measurement. In describing them to you, I will use a few anatomical terms for the sake of precision. If you will examine your hand, you will see that each finger is built of three segments, called *phalanges,* while your thumb has only two. The anatomical terms for the phalanges are:

Distal: the outer phalange—the one bearing the fingernail or thumbnail.

Middle: the next one in. The thumb has no middle phalange.

Proximal: The inner one—the finger segment on which you might wear a ring.

Now look at the drawings. They illustrate the two variable measurements commonly used in acupuncture and auto-acupressure:

Finger width: the width of one proximal phalange.

FIGURE 2

FIGURE 3

FIGURE 4

Finger inch: the width of the distal phalange of the thumb. Or—an alternate way to arrive at it—the distance between the two creases or folds in the middle of your middle finger: the creases at the two ends of the middle phalange.

Four finger widths should equal roughly three finger inches. Check this with your own hands, using both methods of finding the finger inch. With one hand stretched out flat, fingers together, use the other hand to mark off three finger inches across the four proximal phalanges. You may find that the four-to-three ratio works out more precisely with one method of measuring the finger inch than with the other. If so, abandon the less accurate method.

These variable measurements are not accurate to the last millimeter. But they will help you find the approximate locations of the pressure points. Once you are probing near a point, you will usually be able to locate it quickly by being alert to the special sensation of tenderness. When you feel that sensation, it is the signal that your thumbnail has hit the point precisely.

The illustrations and directions that follow should guide you to the approximate location of each point. From there, it will be simply a matter of probing with your thumbnails until you hit the target.

CHAPTER 16

Relieving Back Pains with the Auto-Acupressure System of Body Points: The Knee Points

POINT KNEE 1

Chinese Name: Liang-Ch'iu

English Translation: Beam Mound

Comments: *Point Knee 1* is among the easiest points to reach, and it often signals its location by being exceptionally tender. Those are two reasons why I have chosen to start with it. Moreover, this point may be the only body point many people will need to stimulate. It is especially effective in relieving back pain that travels into the thigh.

Location: The point is exactly two finger widths above the upper, outer border of the kneecap or patella (see Fig. 5). There is a small depression at this spot. Dig your thumbnail hard into the depression, and you should feel a peculiar sensation traveling up your thigh.

If you have trouble locating it, try the following approach. Sit down, with left leg straight, and rest your right palm on your left kneecap as shown in Fig. 6.

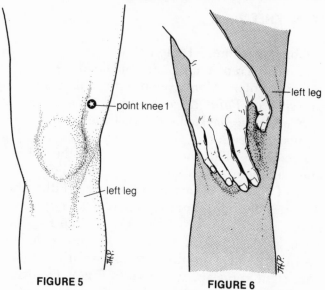

point knee 1

left leg

left leg

FIGURE 5   **FIGURE 6**

Point Knee 1 will be approximately where your bent thumbtip rests. To find the matching point above the other knee, of course, you reverse the procedure.

Stimulation: *Point Knee 1* is stimulated by pressing the fingers into the underside of the thigh. Bend your thumb and press the thumbnail into *Point Knee 1,* as is shown in Fig. 7.

left leg

FIGURE 7

POINT KNEE 2

Chinese Name: Hsueh-Hai

English Translation: Sea of Blood

Comments: Many people find that simultaneous pressure on *Point Knee 1* and *Point Knee 2* produces very effective backache relief. In many cases, no other points are needed.

Location: This point is on the other side of the kneecap from *Point Knee 1*, on the medial or inward side of the leg. Exactly two finger widths above the upper, inner border of the kneecap is a depression, and in that depression lies *Point Knee 2* (see Fig. 8).

To guide yourself to the approximate location, sit down as before, but this time put your right palm over your right kneecap, as shown in Fig. 9. *Point Knee 2* is roughly where your bent thumbtip rests.

This point, too, is often exquisitely tender during backache episodes. You may find it highly sensitive at other times as well. Many people are quite ticklish

FIGURE 8   **FIGURE 9**

point knee 2

point knee 1

left leg

FIGURE 10

when clutched simultaneously at the *Point Knee 1* and *Point Knee 2* locations.

Stimulation: The two points can be simultaneously stimulated in auto-acupressure too. Use both thumbnails first on one knee, then on the other. Fig. 10 shows how to exert maximum thumbnail pressure on these two points. Wrap your fingers under your thigh and squeeze.

POINT KNEE 3

Chinese Name: Wei-Chung
English Translation: Commanding Median
Comments: *Point Knee 3* is especially useful for relieving pains in the thigh and calf. As with the other knee points, it may be the only body point that you need to stimulate.

FIGURE 11   FIGURE 12

Location: The point is behind the knee. It is exactly in the middle of the popliteal transverse crease, the fold at the back of your knee joint (see Fig. 11). Like the other two knee loci, *Point Knee 3* is often sensitive. You can find it by probing along the popliteal crease with your thumbnail until you hit a spot that sends odd sensations shooting down your leg.

Stimulation: This locus is easy to stimulate. Some people find it more natural to stimulate the right locus with the right hand, the left with the left. Others find that they feel more comfortable crossing over and stimulating each point with the opposite-sided hand. Either way, your fingers should be on the front of your leg, knee bent, just below the knee (Fig. 12), to help your bent thumb apply the necessary force.

If you wish, you can reinforce one hand with the other. Or, if you find that you can obtain good results with just one-handed pressure, you can stimulate both *Point Knee 3* points simultaneously.

CHAPTER **17**

Relieving Back Pains with the Auto-Acupressure System of Body Points: The Ankle Point

THE ANKLE POINT

Chinese Name: K'un-lun

English Translation: K'un Lun Mountains

Comments: *The Ankle Point* is especially effective in relieving back pains that radiate down the leg. In combination with *Point Thigh 1* (or with *Points Thigh 1* and *2*, see Figs. 20–24), it may be the only body point you need to stimulate. Some people will find that just stimulating *The Ankle Point* provides sufficient pain relief for leg and back pains.

Location: This point is on the outer side of your ankle. The large bony protuberance there, the lower end of the fibula or outer leg bone, is called the lateral malleolus. Rearward from the malleolus, between it and the heel cord (the calcaneus or Achilles tendon), is a large, almost bowl-shaped depression. *The Ankle Point* is in that depression, precisely in its center, at the same level as the tip of the lateral malleolus (see Fig. 13).

the ankle point

right foot

FIGURE 13

Stimulation: There are two ways to stimulate this point. Some people find they can exert effective pressure by putting the fingers under the heel (Fig. 14). Most, however, seem to get stronger action with the fingers around the back of the heel cord and behind the inner side of the ankle (see Fig. 15).

right foot

right foot

FIGURE 14   **FIGURE 15**

CHAPTER **18**

Relieving Back Pains with the Auto-Acupressure System of Body Points: The Back Points

POINT BACK 1

Chinese Name: Ta Ch'ang Shu
English Translation: Large Intestine Locus
Comments: It is possible to use *Point Back 1* in public without drawing attention to yourself. Using the hands-on-hips technique, the points can be stimulated while the person appears quite natural. It is an excellent point to use to alleviate back strain while sitting.
Location: This is among the more difficult points for most people to locate, so you may need to do somewhat more probing than was necessary with the easily found knee and ankle points. Remember to be alert for the phenomenon of "traveling" sensation that lets you know you are on target. If you have trouble finding the point, it may make its presence known more clearly when you next suffer from backache.

The point (Fig. 16) is in the lumbar region of the back, 1½ finger inches out from the center of the spine on each side. If you run your fingers up your spine, the

4th lumbar vertebra

point back 1

FIGURE 16

bony knobs that you feel are the rearward-projecting spinous processes of the vertebrae. The tips of the spinous processes mark the exact center of the back.

Measuring sideways 1½ finger inches from the spinous processes will help you fix the lateral position of *Point Back 1*. Finding the vertical position will be harder.

The point is near the spinous process of the fourth lumbar vertebra. It is slightly lower than the top of the ilium with the thumbs extending horizontally back toward the spine, as shown in Fig. 17. The *Back 1* pair of points should be roughly where your thumbtips rest. Probe the area until you find a small depression, remembering not to go closer to your spine than a finger inch and a half. *Point Back 1* is in the depression and, like other points, should be noticeably sensitive when you apply thumbnail pressure to it.

Stimulation: The *Back 1* points can be stimulated simultaneously on both sides. The same position used

FIGURE 17

in finding the point can be used to stimulate it. Most people find that the hands-on-hips position allows for strong, sustained pressure.

POINT BACK 2

Chinese Name: Huan-T'iao
English Translation: Circular Jump
Comments: *Point Back 2* is highly effective for relieving sciatic pain. Some people may find that this point alone is sufficient for relief from sciatica.
Location: This point is lower on the back than *Point Back 1*. It is found at the top of the buttocks. As Fig. 18 shows, it is in between the sacrum (the bone that anchors the spine into the pelvic girdle) and the greater trochanter (the large knob near the upper end of the thighbone).
To find this point, you must first find the greater tro-

point back 1

FIGURE 18

chanter. The ilium is the hipbone. It is the top and side of the pelvic girdle, the great bone on which your belt rests. The greater trochanter is a good deal lower.

Stand up and put the heel of your hand on your hipbone, with the fingers extending straight down the side of your leg. Move your leg back and forth and from side to side. You should feel a large, round bony knob moving under your fingertips. That is the greater trochanter. This great bony protuberance is on the outer side of the thighbone (femur). It is slightly below the point where the rounded end, or head, of the femur fits into its hip socket.

To find *Point Back 2*, lie down on your left side with your knees drawn up comfortably. Do not cramp your knees against your chest. Find the greater trochanter with your fingers. Then slide your thumb around your back until you find your sacrum; it is the large, flat prominence between the base of the spine and the tailbone. In most people, the outline of the sacrum is fairly easy to feel. If you have trouble, you may find the sacrum more easily by moving your hips. The sacroiliac joint is not very flexible. However, it is sometimes possible to feel some movement between the sacrum and the pelvic bone on either side.

FIGURE 19

Now estimate the distance between the trochanter and the nearest edge of the sacrum. *Point Back 2* is closer to the trochanter, about one-third of the distance from that bony knob to the sacrum.

Stimulation: *Point Back 2* is stimulated by wrapping the fingers around the thighbone (femur). The hand is extended and the bent thumb is positioned to apply pressure to *Point Back 2* (Fig. 19).

CHAPTER **19**

Relieving Back Pains with the Auto-Acupressure System of Body Points: The Thigh Points

POINT THIGH 1

Chinese Name: Fung-Shih
English Translation: Windy Fair
Comments: *Point Thigh 1* can be stimulated without appearing unnatural, if you are seated at a desk or table. It is also a convenient point to stimulate for back pain that occurs while seated.
Location: On the outside of your thigh is a long "valley" between two large muscles, the biceps femoris and the vastus lateralis. *Point Thigh 1* is in that valley on the outside of the thigh. It is 7 finger inches higher than the popliteal crease at the back of the knee (Fig. 20).

An easy way for most people to locate it is to stand at attention with your hands flat against the outsides of your thighs. *Point Thigh 1* will be near the tip of each middle finger (Fig. 21).
Stimulation: Once you find it and are sure of its

vastus lateralis

biceps femoris ——————⊕———— point thigh 1

point thigh 1

FIGURE 20   **FIGURE 21**

location, you may find you can stimulate it most easily with your bent thumbs while seated. The point can be pressed bilaterally with the fingers wrapped around the under surface of the thighs for extra leverage (Fig. 22).

FIGURE 22

POINT THIGH 2

Chinese Name: Cheng-Fu
English Translation: Support
Comments: *Point Thigh 2* is one of the very easiest to find. It is also, for many people, one of the most effective for relief of back pain that travels into the buttock.
Location: It is exactly in the middle of the gluteal fold, the crease under the buttocks at the back of each thigh (Fig. 23).
Stimulation: Most people find it easiest to stimulate *Point Thigh 2* one side at a time. Lie on your side. Press the upper point with the upper thumbnail (Fig. 24). If you are lying on your right side, press the point under the left buttock with the thumb of your left hand. Your fingers should be on the upper portion of the buttock.

point thigh 2

left leg

FIGURE 23   FIGURE 24

CHAPTER **20**

Relieving Back Pains with the Auto-Acupressure System of Body Points: The Lower Leg Point

THE LOWER LEG POINT

Chinese Name: Ch'eng-Shan
English Translation: Supporting Hill
Comments: *The Lower Leg Point* is easy to find and easy to stimulate. It is particularly effective for sciatic pain that radiates down into the leg.
Location: The back of your lower leg, or calf, is shaped by a long muscle called the gastrocnemius. It is anchored by the Achilles tendon at its lower end, and above that it divides into two bands of "heads." You can feel a groove between the two heads, precisely in the middle of your calf at its widest point. If you have trouble locating the groove, stand on tiptoe to tense the muscle.

The Lower Leg Point is at the lower end of the muscle groove, 8 finger inches below the popliteal (knee) crease (Fig. 25).

145

FIGURE 25   FIGURE 26

Stimulation: The locus can be stimulated on both sides at one time. Put the nail of your bent thumb in the point, and apply opposing pressure with your fingers on your shinbone (Fig. 26).

Relieving Back Pains with the Auto-Acupressure System of Body Points: A Review

If you have studied the last five chapters, you have learned how to locate and stimulate nine pairs of body points. As we explained in Chapter 10, most people find it necessary to stimulate only one or two body points, or pairs of body points. Many people will now find it helpful to review the basic principles of relieving back pains that we discussed in Chapter 10. Those include the following:

1. Preparation before starting auto-acupressure
   a. Diagnosis of problem
   b. Reevaluation of drug regimens
2. The thumbnail technique
3. Use of muscle leverage
4. Amount of pressure necessary
5. How long to press
6. Choosing auto-acupressure points
   a. Which are most effective
   b. Which are easiest to stimulate
7. Pairing of points
8. Repeat applications
9. Body position during point stimulation

When you feel that you have a working knowledge of the system of body points, you are ready to learn about the ear point system. Many people find that stimulating a single ear point, or pair of ear points, brings relief from back pains. Others may find that stimulating the combination of a single ear point and a single body point produces quick and significant relief from back pains.

In the next chapter, we will study the basic principles of relieving back pains with the auto-acupressure system of ear points.

CHAPTER **22**

Relieving Back Pains with the Auto-Acupressure System of Ear Points: Basic Principles

Western medical researchers and Oriental acupuncturists have observed a highly consistent pattern of connections between various points in the ears and corresponding body parts. Every part of the body is represented: the head, the trunk, the limbs and extremities. It is possible to draw a schematic map of the entire body in the two pinnae; it would show that certain parts of the ears contain neural connections with the hands, certain parts with the hips, and so on. This tracery of nerves in the ears is a miniaturized reflection of certain nerve pathways in the body as a whole.

The existence of such a convenient ear point system is one good reason for attacking a backache through the ears. Another reason is that the nerves of the ear point system are peculiarly accessible to thumbnail pressure. The external ears are built mainly of thin cartilage covered with skin. They ordinarily contain no bone, and most parts of the ear contain no muscle. In many other parts of the body, nerves are often hidden behind bone or buried in deep masses of muscle and other tissue. There is no convenient way to stimulate them. However, in the pinnae, the nerves are easily accessible for stimulation.

The ear point system can be used before, after, or in conjunction with the body point system, or the ear point system can be used alone. Many people find that the ear point system gives them excellent relief most of the time. They use the body point system less often; sometimes, only when their pain is more than usually severe. Others find that certain combinations of the two systems work best for them.

I suggest that you experiment in the following way when you are next troubled by a backache. Try the ear point system first. If it gives you only partial relief, try those body points that you have found to be the most effective for you.

That combination may give you effective, long-lasting relief. However, some people find that reversing the combination works better for them. They use the body point system for *initial* relief, as at the beginning of an arduous day. Then use the ear point system for *maintenance* of the effects throughout the day.

An advantage of the ear point system is that you can use it at any time of day. You can use it in any situation, in public or in private. Some of the body point system points require that you partially undress, lie down, or adopt somewhat awkward positions. Consequently, it is not always possible to stimulate some of the body points in the middle of a busy day. Some of those points can be pressed unobtrusively while sitting in a chair, but others cannot. Thus you may find the ear point system highly useful. If a backache is troubling you while you are at work, at a social gathering, or riding in a car, you can stimulate the ear points quite unobtrusively. To other people, you will look as though you are only toying with your ears, a perfectly natural human gesture. (Your thumbnail may leave a red mark. However, it should not be very noticeable and should vanish in minutes.)

STIMULATION

In stimulating the ear points, be guided in general by the directions I gave in Chapter 10, dealing with the body point system. The stimulation techniques for both systems are substantially the same.

Use your thumbnail, with the thumb bent as shown in Fig. 1, page 128. With most points, to give the thumbnail something to press against, you can put your forefinger on the other side of the ear for a pincerlike squeezing action. Press hard enough to make the point under your thumbnail hurt mildly. As with the body point system, you can use either steady pressure or rhythmic off–on pressure. Maintain it for 30 seconds.

As I warned before, it is dangerous to apply auto-acupressure with long or pointed thumbnails. The nails should be short and rounded. It is never necessary in auto-acupressure to pierce the skin or to leave any injury beyond a temporary red mark.

WHICH EAR?

If your back pain is centered or diffuse, not clearly one-sided, then you will generally find it most effective to press paired points on both ears.

If the pain is one-sided, one ear may well be sufficient. Often, in the case of one-sided pain, you will find that certain points on one ear are markedly more tender than the corresponding points on the other ear. Do not assume, however, that the tender ear will always be on the same side of the body as the back, buttock, or leg pain. Under some circumstances, you will find that the opposite-sided ear is the more tender.

Thus, when your back pains, you will need to explore your ears for tenderness. As with the body point system, the greatest pain-relieving effect always comes from stimulating the most tender points.

CHAPTER **23**

Relieving Back Pains with the Auto-Acupressure System of Ear Points: Structure of the Ear

In medical terminology, the external ear is called the auricula or pinna. It is richly endowed with a highly complex network of fine but amazingly sensitive nerves. They interconnect through many neural pathways with nerves in distant parts of the body. When they are stimulated properly with either a needle or a thumbnail, they can produce astonishingly powerful effects in those distant parts. You are soon to discover the effects on pain in the back, the buttocks, and the legs.

In the next chapter, with words and drawings, I will guide you through the ear point system. You will learn points that are relevant to back pains and to the sciatic pains and leg pains that are often their unwelcome companion. But first, as we did with the body point system, I will need to give you some instruction on basic anatomy.

EXPLORING YOUR EARS

If you will study your ears in a mirror, you will probably see that they are not shaped precisely alike. In

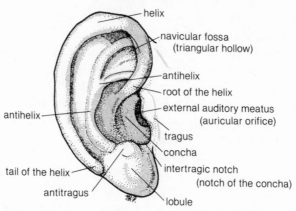

helix

navicular fossa
(triangular hollow)

antihelix

root of the helix

external auditory meatus
(auricular orifice)

antihelix

tragus

concha

tail of the helix

intertragic notch
(notch of the concha)

antitragus

lobule

FIGURE 27

some people, the difference is immediately apparent, while in others, it is subtle: a more pronounced curve here, a longer groove there. Ears are remarkably variable, even on the same head.

They are still more variable from one person to another. The size, the degree of protrusion, the color, the shapes of various parts of the structure vary wildly. This is even true in members of the same family.

The ear changes shape and texture continually through life. A child's ear cartilage is soft and very pliable. As he ages, it will grow harder and less elastic. Some parts may wrinkle; the lobe may grow longer; hair may appear on the top and elsewhere. If the ear has been subjected to a lot of trauma in its lifetime, there may be some fairly gross changes and distortions. The "cauliflower ear" of a boxer is an exaggerated example. Ears that have been frequently exposed to severe cold or to sunburn may also become more than normally thickened.

But despite all these variations, the basic design of the human pinna remains constant from one head to another. If you will look at Fig. 27, you will see a drawing of an ear with the prominent parts named. You will need to know the names of these parts to follow the directions in the next chapter. Study the drawing and identify the parts on your own ears by exploring them with thumb and forefinger. There are not many of them. Some of the names are appealingly imaginative. To help you in your exploration, I will supplement the drawing by describing the parts in words:

The large central cavity is called the *concha,* from a Greek word meaning seashell.

The ear-canal hole in the concha is called the *auricular orifice* or the *external auditory meatus* (pronounced me-ay-tus).

Directly in front of the meatus and partly covering it is a prominent little knob of cartilage called the *tragus.* In some people the tragus has, on its underside, a tuft of hair something like a goat's beard. The name literally means he-goat.

Across the concha from the tragus, and separated from it by a small notch, is another outcropping of cartilage called the *antitragus.* The notch is called the *intertragic notch* or simply the *notch of the concha.*

Below the antitragus is the lobe; in medical terminology it is called the *lobule.* It contains no cartilage. From ancient times, it has been used by both men and women as a place from which to hang rings and other decorations. In some people, the lobe is securely attached to the neighboring facial skin near the angle of the jaw. In others it is clearly separate. This is an oddity of heredity and is linked to certain other inherited traits.

The prominent outer rim of the ear is called the *helix.* Follow it on your own ear with thumb and finger and you will notice that it starts just above the lobe. This is the so-called *tail* of the helix. The helix then runs up the side of the ear, over the top, and down into the concha. This part of the helix, where it runs backward across the bowl of the concha, is called the *root* or *crus* (rhymes with "loose"). The crus of the helix divides the concha into two unequal parts.

Inside the helix, running parallel with it for a short distance, is another ridge called the *antihelix*. Toward the top of the ear the antihelix divides into two ridges or *crura*. Both ridges then disappear under the helix. Between these two crura is a shallow triangular depression which is named the *navicular fossa*. *Navicular* means boat-shaped, and *fossa* comes from a word meaning ditch. For simplicity, I will refer to this area from now on as the *triangular hollow*.

Now, while you remember the basic structure of the external ear, it is the time to learn how to relieve back pains with the ear point system.

CHAPTER **24**

Relieving Back Pains with the Auto-Acupressure System of Ear Points: Methods of Location and Stimulation

To find these points, you will have to use, in miniature, a technique you learned in Chapter 14. Each point has a peculiarly tender feeling, and when you feel it, that is the signal that you are on target. As we go through the points, I will describe each as closely as I can. You should also refer to Fig. 26 for further guidance. But the final targeting will be up to you. Put your thumbnail in the approximate location of each point; then move it back and forth, by the smallest possible increments, until you touch the tender spot for which you are looking.

If you have trouble finding the points under ordinary conditions, wait until your next attack of back pain. It is likely that some, or all, of the points will then become considerably more tender.

THE STARTING POINT

As Fig. 28 shows, this is on the root or crus of the helix as it exits from the concha. In many people, there is a fairly deep crosswise notch in the crus at this point, much like a notch in a long mountain ridge. Other people will find a tiny knob of cartilage just behind the point. Probe with your thumbnail until you feel this often tender spot. During episodes of back pain, it may become exquisitely tender.

It is called the *Starting Point* because it is probably the easiest of all microsystem points to find. You may want to experiment with it before going on to the other points. Stimulating this point may produce excellent relief of lumbar and sciatic pain. Some people find that it is usually the only microsystem point they need.

Some find that they can stimulate this point well by putting the forefinger behind the ear and squeezing against the thumbnail. In most people, however, the ear is attached to the head in such a way that it is hard to get the forefinger into the right position. If you find that this is the case with you, stimulate the point by pressing directly inward against your head (Fig. 29).

FIGURE 28

FIGURE 29   FIGURE 30

THE ANTIHELIX LOW BACK POINTS

The positions of these points vary from person to person and from time to time in the same person, depending on the exact nature and location of the back disorder. As Fig. 28 shows, the *Antihelix Low Back Points* lie along the lower ridge of the antihelix, starting at the place where the two ridges form a fork (the apex of the triangular hollow) and ending where the lower ridge disappears under the overlying helix.

When you have pain in the lower back or sacroiliac area, probe along that antihelix ridge with your thumbnail until you find the most tender point. Start by lifting the overlying helix and probing under it. Then very slowly work your way back to the fork of the antihelix.

To stimulate this point effectively, form pincers with your thumb and forefinger. The thumbnail should press directly into the point on the outer surface of your ear, while the fingernail presses the same point from behind (Fig. 30).

THE TRIANGULAR HOLLOW POINTS

Points relating to the lower back are in the lower, rearward part of the triangular hollow. They are near the fork of the two antihelix ridges (see Fig. 28). As

FIGURE 31

before, you should probe with your thumbnail in very small increments until you find unusual tenderness.

These points, when well stimulated, relieve pain and spasm in the region of the sacroiliac, the buttocks, and the thighs. They can be stimulated effectively with the thumb-and-forefinger pincers (Fig. 31).

THE ANTIHELIX MID-BACK POINTS

These points are on the antihelix, at or above the place where the crus of the helix abuts against it. When stimulated correctly, a tender point in this area relieves pain and spasm in the thoracic or mid-back region (Fig. 28).

The point can be stimulated, like the others, with the thumbnail on the outer ear surface and the nail of the forefinger behind it.

THE TRAGUS POINT

Use this point for chronic back pain if you fail to get adequate relief from the points we have already studied. As Fig. 28 shows, the point is near the top and toward the front of the tragus. It is just behind the place

FIGURE 32

(marked on some people by a faint groove) where the tragus joins the side of the face. In most people, the point is directly in front of the meatus (the opening of the ear canal).

This point is unlike all the others in one very important respect. It is never necessary to stimulate the point on both ears. Instead, utilize the following procedure:

If you are right-handed, stimulate the left tragus. If you are left-handed, stimulate the right. This somewhat mysterious-sounding rule is dictated by a peculiarity of the nervous system. The tragus opposite the hand-favored side is always the one with the clearest neural connections with the spine.

Most people find it comfortable to stimulate the *Tragus Point* with the favored hand. That is, if you are right-handed, stimulate the left point with your right hand. Hold the tragus between thumbnail and forefinger so that the thumbnail is vertical. Be careful not to let your forefingernail slip into the ear-canal opening (Fig. 32).

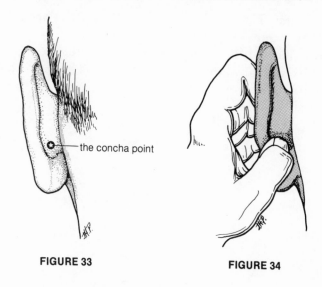

FIGURE 33

the concha point

FIGURE 34

THE CONCHA POINT

This point, unlike the others, is behind the ear rather than on its outer surface. Study its location carefully in Fig. 33.

To find the point, put your forefinger in the concha, just above the intertragus notch. Your thumb should be behind your ear with the pad of the thumb resting against the back of the lobe. With the tip of your thumb, you will feel a convex bowl of cartilage, the underside of the concha. Now probe with your thumbnail near the lower, inner corner of the cartilage, close to the lobe and close to the place where the ear joins the neck. You should find an extremely tender point there, particularly during episodes of lower back pain (Fig. 34).

The point corresponds to the lower part of the spine. Many people find it highly effective when used after one of the *Antihelix Low Back Points*.

Once you have learned to locate and stimulate the ear points, you should select your favorite point or two. During your next episode of back pain, try the ear point system first. Then try it in combination with your favorite body point.

Now that you know how to relieve your back pains, it is wise to learn how to prevent them. The next chapter will advise you on how to live with a back that is vulnerable to pain.

25

Living with Our Vulnerable Backs

A vulnerable back is one that is subject to frequent or chronic pain. As we saw in Chapters 5, 6, and 7, there are a variety of possible reasons for such pain. In Chapters 7 and 8, we reviewed the use of drugs for back pains. Then in Chapters 10–21, we learned how to relieve back pains with the Auto-Acupressure Systems of Body Points and Ear Points. This chapter will advise you on other precautionary measures to reduce the frequency and severity of painful episodes.

EXERCISE

This is one topic on which you should most certainly consult your doctor. Certain exercises can aggravate a back problem instead of alleviating it. That is why I do not intend to prescribe exercises in this book. Only a doctor who is familiar with your entire health status will know whether a given exercise would be beneficial, dangerous, or useless to you.

In most cases, people with vulnerable backs are encouraged to exercise daily so as to strengthen muscles of the abdomen, the back, and the buttocks. These are the muscle areas that do the major work of holding the spine erect and maintaining the proper curvatures. If you allow your abdominal muscles to become weak, the ultimate result could be a protruding abdomen that might produce a sway-backed posture (lordosis) which will put damaging stress on the lumbar area of your spine. The muscles of the back itself do the main work of supporting the upper part of the spine. The large buttock muscles help hold the upper body in proper alignment with hips and legs.

In many cases, a physician will suggest calisthenics such as bent-knee and pelvic-tilt sit-ups, designed to demand strenuous exertion of certain specific muscle groups. However, such exercises are hard work and are boring. The unfortunate truth is that only a minority of people actually perform them religiously over a span of years. Thus, many doctors simply counsel back patients to get plenty of general exercise in some activity they enjoy, such as swimming, walking, bicycling, etc. It can certainly be stated as a general truth that your chances of avoiding back problems grow very much better as you improve your muscle tone and strength, your posture, and other aspects of your general health.

BODY WEIGHT

Try to keep your weight within the normal tolerances for a man or woman of your height. It is obvious that a heavy upper body will put more than normal stress on the spine as it tries to hold all that weight upright.

But if you are now overweight, beware of fad dieting or any attempt to shed pounds in too great a hurry. As we saw in an earlier chapter, poor nutrition can aggravate certain back disorders. It can even become one of their basic causes. There are safe and unsafe ways to lose weight. In your local library, you will find books devoted to both ways. Ask your doctor to recommend one of the safe ones.

SITTING

Favor straight-backed, firm chairs, not heavily padded ones. The body sinks too deeply into thick pad-
ding, causing excessive flexure of the spine.

When you sit, try to have one or both knees higher
than your hips. This is the sitting position that puts the
least strain on the spine. Crossing your legs will lift one
knee high. Or you can lift both knees by putting your
feet on a low stool. However, be sure your knees are
bent, so that your feet rest on their soles. Do not extend
your legs straight out so that your feet rest on the backs
of the heels. That position increases strain on the back.

To improve your sitting posture when driving a car,
pull the seat forward enough to lift your knees high.
When riding as a passenger, cross your legs or put one
foot on the transmission hump. You may find that car
seats are too deeply padded for you, and that you develop pain and stiffness on trips that are not especially
long. If so, you may get relief from a special straight-
backed car seat. Such seats are made to fit over the
standard padded seats. They can be bought at medical
supply houses and some department stores.

UNUSUALLY HEAVY STRESS

You may know in advance that you must endure a
particularly stressful day. For example, you must take a
long automobile trip and then unload heavy suitcases
from the car. You know from past experience that this
will produce back pain. In a case such as this, ask your
doctor beforehand if he can recommend temporary
help. He may prescribe a back brace or orthopedic cor-
set. Such a device can help you through a period of
unusually heavy back stress. In these special situations,
it may help you avoid new back damage.

An orthopedic appliance such as a back brace should be looked upon only as a temporary aid. Remove it as soon as you and your physician feel it is safe to do so. You should beware of becoming dependent on it. If you lapse into the habit of wearing it every day, you could dangerously weaken your back and the muscles that support it.

CAR DOORS

One very common body movement that can cause pain, and even acute trauma when awkwardly done, is that of climbing in and out of a car. The action of ducking the head while twisting the body is hard to carry out gracefully.

A good procedure is to get in and out of the car much as you would get in and out of bed. When entering the car, first sit sideways on the edge of the seat, with your feet outside on the ground. Then lean back so that your head clears the doorway and enters the car. Finally, swing your legs inside. To climb out, reverse the process: first swing your feet sideways and out onto the ground, and then lean forward enough to stand.

STANDING

If you must stand still for a long time, try to rest one foot higher than the other. If you are working on a ladder, put one foot on a rung higher than the other. If you are waiting at an airport or railroad station, rest one foot on your suitcase.

This standing position puts the least possible strain on the back. Tavernkeepers all over the world are aware of this. At almost any bar where the patrons stand, there is a rail on which they can rest one foot. Utilizing the bar rail with occasional changes in position, many people find it is possible to stand for several hours without discomfort. By contrast, an uncomfortable experience for most back pain sufferers is a cocktail party where one must spend a long time standing with both feet flat on the floor. In such situations, you will probably find it helpful to straighten the back while standing. You can do so by tilting the pelvis. To further reduce strain, bend one knee, and keep the other knee straight.

BENDING AND LIFTING

When you bend to pick something up, you should bend your knees as well as your back. If the object is heavy, make your legs do most of the work.

If you carry a heavy weight for any distance, carry it close to your body with your elbows bent, not straight. Even with bent elbows, it is hazardous to lift a heavy weight higher than shoulder level. If you are carrying some heavy or awkward object with another person, be sure that both of you lift it and put it down together, as a team. If the other person drops his or her end, drop yours too. Trying to catch a heavy weight in that manner can do serious damage to your back. It is better to break a piece of furniture than a vertebra.

When carrying anything heavy, do not twist your body. If you must turn while heavily burdened, turn with your feet.

Avoid lifting heavy objects that are in tight, awkward places. Be especially careful with objects so situated that you cannot get your feet under the weight. You will recall that I injured my own back once when trying to lift a sack of lawn fertilizer from a car trunk. The standard car trunk could hardly have been more ineptly designed; it is hard to think of anything harder on the spine. If you must remove anything heavy from a car trunk or any similarly awkward space, either get help or roll the object out. If at all possible, avoid lifting it out.

If you must bend down to pick up something, it is wise to avoid bending with your knees straight. It will be easier on your back either to crouch down on both legs or rest on one knee only. When working with something on the ground, it is better to bend down on one knee rather than on both.

SLEEPING

People with low back pain generally should not lie on their stomachs. For the sake of your back, lie on your side with knees and hips bent. Or lie on your back with a pillow (or rolled blanket or other object) under your knees to bend the knees and hips.

It is best to use a firm, flat mattress. Try to avoid a soft, deep mattress, or an old one with a depression in the middle. Your bed should not allow the middle of your body to sag as in a hammock; it should support your hips firmly, with just enough softness for comfort. If your bed is too soft, you can get relief by putting a bedboard under the mattress.

When traveling, you can get a bedboard on request at many hotels and motels. If that is not possible and if a hotel bed is too soft, make arrangements for someone else to take the mattress off the box spring and put it on the floor. Or you can simply spread blankets on the floor and sleep on them.

FATIGUE

It is best to avoid getting excessively tired during the day. Fatigue can exacerbate many low back problems.

When I was a medical student, I was puzzled one day to see an obstetrician squatting in a crouched position in a hospital corridor. He saw my perplexed look, smiled, and explained that he did this periodically to ease the strain on his back. His work often required him to stand for long periods, bending over an operating table. The squatting position made him feel better in a few minutes.

Anybody with a vulnerable back would do well to emulate that man. Try to find a way of relaxing your back for 5 or 10 minutes, once or twice a day. If possible, lie flat on your back on a bed or floor. Elevate your legs on a pillow or cushion so as to exert a mild upward pull on the hips. If you feel pain, you can relieve it with auto-acupressure.

CHAPTER **26**

Relaxation Techniques: Rest Without Pills

Most chronic back pain patients rely on some sort of drug to assist sleep. In a recent study at the Mayo Clinic, 65 percent of patients with chronic pain, not related to malignant tumors, were found to be either drug dependent or drug abusers. In addition to analgesics, tranquilizers, and muscle relaxants, many of my patients have related prior abuse of sleeping pills and alcoholic beverages to induce sleep. Furthermore, many patients have related to me that they had persistent difficulties with insomnia even after they had learned to relieve their back pains with auto-acupressure. They expressed dissatisfaction with their dependence on pills for sleep, and wanted to "kick the habit" of drugs for sleep.

The solution I ordinarily offer for such problems involves tapering off unnecessary drugs and substituting a relaxation technique. The brain must sleep. Once pain problems are brought under control, it is ordinarily the inability to relax that delays the onset of sleep.

Because of their sedative effects, relaxation techniques are excellent methods to augment pain relief systems. Being overanxious, being uptight often causes intensification of both muscle spasm and the subjective discomfort of pain. The more a person's focus turns to the inner awareness of pain, the greater may be the dread of possible destructive effects of pain upon the ability to enjoy and participate in life. Ordinarily, the awareness of pain increases suffering. But there are exceptions. The often quoted observation of wounded soldiers in the battlefield relates the fact that what might otherwise be excruciating pain can be perceived in a positive way. Soldiers with severe wounds have been seen to exhibit euphoria at having earned "their ticket back home." In these days of relative cold rather than hot wars, there are many ferocious "battles" conducted on athletic fields. It is certainly well known and well documented that sometimes professional and non-professional athletes have played with serious injuries. They were able to overcome pain in the desire for victory.

My acquaintance with relaxation techniques dates back more than three decades ago when I learned techniques of hypnosis. I had the good fortune to witness the use of hypnosis in the treatment of various habit disorders. I was instructed by an excellent hypnotist, who had the ability to induce hypnotic trances in a variety of people. Over two-and-a-half decades ago, I wrote my first monograph on the induction of hypnosis and self-hypnosis. I mention these points to emphasize that I have been able to observe the long-term effectiveness of these techniques over a considerable period of time.

Hypnosis is a state of altered consciousness. It is a condition of heightened awareness of certain stimuli and decreased awareness of others. Hypnosis is better suited for relief of acute pain situations than of chronic pain situations. The use of hypnosis as both an analgesic and an anesthetic agent has been well documented. Surgical operations have been conducted using hypnosis as the primary anesthetic.

Currently, I utilize hypnosis in my private office practice for the following special effects: (1) overcoming memory blocks and resistances in the course of psychotherapy, (2) weight reduction, (3) smoking reduction, and (4) insomnia problems.

Posthypnotic suggestions may alter a person's behavior after the cessation of the formal hypnotic state. Posthypnotic suggestions are utilized in the hypnotic treatment techniques for weight reduction and smoking control. In those cases, the posthypnotic suggestions given are ordinarily positive ones which encourage the development of aversions to the specific appetites. The treatment of chronic pain may be attempted with a negative posthypnotic suggestion, such as the absence of awareness. Since denying the awareness of pain is unrealistic, it is not usually a successful method. Positive posthypnotic suggestions are sometimes beneficial for pain relief. Some patients do respond to associating the perception of pain with pleasant memories and sensations. Again, however, these effects tend to be transient. Ordinarily, they do not produce substantial long-term benefit in most chronic pain patients.

The use of self-hypnosis in insomnia problems is quite helpful for some patients. Nevertheless, it is not a technique which I feel is appropriate for everyone. It requires consultation from a psychiatrist to determine whether self-hypnosis is a desirable procedure. However, a closely related relaxation technique to assist in producing sleep will be offered to you—in detail—at the conclusion of this short chapter. Many patients have fallen asleep in my office just in the process of learning it.

Biofeedback is a relaxation technique whereby a person learns to relax muscles which he ordinarily would not have under voluntary control. Biofeedback is a meritorious technique for patients who can learn to use it. Generally, it provides assistance to chronic pain patients and is one of those techniques which can be used to modify pain. Biofeedback is generally able to decrease the perception of some pains by decreasing painful muscle spasm. There are biofeedback instruments available in professional laboratories and available for home use. Your physician may be able to direct you to someone who can train you in the biofeedback method. Or he may recommend that you buy a biofeedback device to use at home. In brief essence, the biofeedback method would involve the electronic monitoring of a bodily function, such as pulse rate, hand warmth, or muscle movement. If, for example, your low back pain caused spasm in the lumbar muscles, electrodes might be attached to those muscles. You could work with the machine until you had developed a state of relaxation in the muscles. Ideally then, you might be able to learn to sit or stand with the same degree of relaxation of your low back muscles as you might obtain at other times when you are lying flat on your back with a pillow under your knees.

Although it was felt that biofeedback might be an answer to many pain problems, long-term follow-up studies simply have not shown that to be the case. Even though one's expectations should be limited, it is again emphasized that this may be a helpful supplementary technique and its use should be considered on advice of your personal physician.

Much wisdom about relaxation may be found in the study of yoga. However, the advice of your physician should be obtained to determine what hatha yoga exercises are prudent for your general state of health and particular back problems. For more than a half-century, the pioneer American physician in the field of relaxation techniques has been Dr. Edmund Jacobson. His extensive bibliography includes several entire books on progressive relaxation exercises.

As I have already promised, here is the simple relaxaation technique which can facilitate the onset of sleep by diminishing anxieties and muscle spasm. This relaxation technique involves the alternate contraction and relaxation of major groups of muscles related to body parts. One starts at the toes and progresses to the head. An example of this effective muscle relaxation technique would be to contract (bend) each set of muscles for 10 to 15 seconds, and then to feel those muscles relax for an equal period of time. To be specific, the relaxation technique would be: bend your toe muscles for 10 seconds. Feel them relax for 10 seconds. Bend the ankle up for 10 seconds. Relax the ankle for 10 seconds. Contract the calf muscles for 10 seconds. Relax the calf muscles for 10 seconds. Contract the thigh muscles for 10 seconds. Relax the thigh muscles for 10 seconds. Contract the abdominal muscles for 10 seconds. Relax the abdominal muscles for 10 seconds. Make a fist for 10 seconds. Relax the fist for 10 seconds. Bend the wrist up for 10 seconds. Relax the wrist for 10 seconds. Contract the upper arm muscles for 10 seconds. Relax the upper arm muscles for 10 seconds. Shrug the shoulder muscles for 10 seconds. Relax the shoulder muscles for 10 seconds. Tense the neck muscles for 10 seconds. Relax the neck muscles for 10 seconds. Contract the forehead muscles for 10 seconds. Relax the forehead muscles for 10 seconds. Contract the eyelids tightly for 10 seconds. Relax the eyelids for 10 seconds, keeping the eyelids lightly closed. Now feel the state of relaxation that has gone from your toes to your head. Feel the relaxation all the way down the body—from the head to the neck to the shoulder to the arm to the hand to the abdomen to the thigh to the calf to the ankle to the toes.

If performing this relaxation technique has not relaxed you suitably the first time, then repeat it. An alternate technique is to use a longer period of time for each muscle group, such as 15 to 30 seconds. Such relaxation techniques should be encouraged. They are a much healthier, more natural and nontoxic substitute for analgesics, sedative tranquilizers, and sleeping pills.

Our consultation on your back pain problems is now

almost complete. We have discussed the major aspects of learning to live more comfortably with your illness. We have consulted on diagnoses and treatment methods. We have learned new methods of pain relief. We have discussed how to adapt to the demands of daily living. We have briefly reviewed methods of overcoming anxiety and sleeping problems without drugs. In the next chapter, you may learn how to make your sexual life more fulfilling.

CHAPTER 27

Sex and the Back Pain Patient: An X-Rated Consultation

One of the most critical problems for back pain patients is the loss, or the fear of loss, of sexual function. This problem was typified in a recent study of married patients referred to the pain management center of the Mayo Clinic. Almost two-thirds of those patients reported impairment in their sexual satisfaction. They stated that sexual intercourse had decreased both in frequency and in quality. Sexual changes, such as these, are very critical life problems. They frequently contribute to deterioration of the overall marital relationship, often resulting in divorce.

A significant percentage of men and women, who did not have sexual difficulties prior to their pain disorders, developed them consequent to their painful state. Frequently occurring sexual problems are difficulties in becoming sexually aroused and in reaching orgasm. Some chronic pain patients lose all interest in sex.

Medication used for pain relief may decrease libido. Tranquilizers, sedatives, and narcotic analgesics all may reduce sexual drive. Corticosteroids may decrease the response to genital stimulation in both males and females. Moreover, corticosteroids may induce impotence in males.

Until very recently, expressions of sexuality or sexual need in physically handicapped people were seen as unusual, if not perverse. Overcoming a person's handicap by obtaining a job or functioning independently are commonly considered praiseworthy achievements. Such praiseworthiness had rarely extended to socially appropriate sexual activity. To most people, the sexual needs of the handicapped individual are considered to vary from humorous to repulsive.

The sexual needs of the physically disabled and chronic pain patients are not identical to those of people in the ablebodied population. People with physical handicaps and chronic pain problems commonly have sexual needs that are accentuated. Their sexual desires are increased by the constant need to be reassured that their disabilities do not repulse their loved ones. Chronic pain patients and physically disabled people usually have an even greater need than others to prove that their sexual performance can be satisfying.

Medical studies of arthritis patients typify those of all patients with chronic pain problems. Many who have suffered from the severe pain, disfigurement, depression, and prolonged hospitalization associated with arthritis have observed that their sexual relationships became a focus of failure and frustration. As chronic arthritis conditions progressed, close marital relationships often deteriorated. They became guilt laden, overburdened with great emotional strain. Many became devoid of sexual intimacy. Frequently, the results were emotional instability, marital separation, and ultimately divorce.

In the early stages of arthritic disease, women patients with back and hip problems may find that limitation in movement of the hips and other joints makes intercourse painful and therefore unsatisfying. In later stages of arthritic hip disease, traditional positions of intercourse may become impossible. Awareness of the destruction of the body, related to the chronic pain and its resultant depression, may also contribute to the person's loss of sexual function. The loss of sexual pleasure is often the arthritic patient's first significant life loss. It often occurs long before the loss of the ability to walk or the loss of the ability to work.

Low back pain and arthritic involvement of the hips are the disabilities most likely to interfere with sexual pleasure. The degree of disability in women created by limitations of hip movement tends to be much greater than that suffered by men. Limitations in the ability of a woman to move the hip bone, especially if it is two-sided, may prevent penetration by the man. There are usually alternate positions that can be utilized. For most women, rear entry positions are still possible despite hip disease. Fortunately, hip problems in men are unlikely to interfere significantly with the mechanical performance of sexual intercourse.

Sufficient preparation for intercourse may be necessary for patients with the most severe back and arthritic problems. Many need a warm-up period similar to that utilized by athletes. Such people may need to have the application of moist warm heat to affected joints. Warm baths, showers, or compresses help to limber up joints prior to having sexual relations. Many doctors encourage arthritic patients to use such procedures as part of foreplay. When a couple bathes together before sex, they get a mutual application of moist heat. The pleasure of such an experience often enables the forgetting of the medicinal aspect of bathing.

The time of day used for sexual activity may affect the amount of pain experienced. Many patients with osteoarthritis prefer mornings. In rheumatoid arthritis patients, fatigue tends to decrease just before noon and again in mid-afternoon. The majority of patients with arthritis have less stiffness at night, making that the best time for sexual intercourse.

A complete and candid discussion of sexual problems with the patient's physician is absolutely essential.

Until that is accomplished, a person should not decide that sexual intercourse is impossible, whatever the physical handicap. Furthermore, if sexual intercourse is mechanically impossible, the physician may discuss alternate means of obtaining sexual gratification. The real goal of sexual activity is the interpersonal pleasure and the intimacy it can bring to a relationship. There are many alternate methods of sexual gratification that can be utilized, even when sexual intercourse is not physically practical. Such methods include masturbation, fellatio (oral sexual stimulation of the penis) and cunnilingus (oral sexual stimulation of the female genitalia).

Fortunately, however, most back pain patients can utilize varying techniques to successfully engage in and enjoy sexual intercourse. Most men with low back problems can engage in intercourse lying flat on the back, utilizing the position of the man below and the woman above. At other times, the side-to-side position enables normal relations. A woman with low back problems may discover she can have pain-free intercourse by lying flat on her back with her knees supported by a pillow, and straddled by the man in a superior position. Alternately, the woman can be on her back or side with one leg raised enabling the man to make a side penetration. In another variation, the woman can be standing, leaning over a table or bed, allowing the man to make a rear penetration. All these may be comfortable and satisfying positions for women with severe back problems.

Patients should inquire of their physicians about positions for intercourse that are most adaptable for their affected joints. Through their own experience, some people will discover workable positions and such trials should be encouraged. Usually, the physician can recommend positions, such as those just described, that take weight off painful joints. It is also helpful for people to be reassured by their physicians that unfamiliar sexual practices may simply be normal variations and not perversions.

In the past, patients suffering from chronic pain, such as the pain of arthritis, have indicated to their physicians that they felt sexual activity made them feel better. Some even said that the sexual act relieved their pain. Because of this, studies have been conducted to discern the action of sexual activity in chronic pain patients. A recent study was conducted with arthritis patients, all of whom were sexually active. It revealed that their sexual activity not only made these patients feel better, but it also relieved their pain. It is unclear whether the sexual activity, in itself, functions as an analgesic. It may well be that the pain is still there, but after a positive sexual experience, it just does not bother the person quite so much.

If a back pain problem intensifies, or in other ways becomes disturbing during sexual activity, auto-acupressure may provide the solution. Auto-acupressure can ordinarily be utilized during sexual relations to relieve, or eliminate, back pain without disturbing the natural flow of events. Whatever the technique or method being employed, most people can usually find a way to free one or both hands for the brief time necessary to produce back pain relief. Even if the affected person cannot (for whatever psychologic or physical reasons) bring himself (or herself) to utilize auto-acupressure during sexual activities, there are still many alternate methods to obtain relief from back pain, utilizing the auto-acupressure systems.

The sexual partner can apply pressure either to the auto-acupressure body system or ear system of points. Either sexual partner can perform, or assist with, the brief application of a transcutaneous neurostimulator (TENS—see Chapter 14) on an auto-acupressure system body point. Patients have reported that brief stimulation of a body system point with a vibrator (that can be used for genital stimulation) not only relieved their back pain, but also made their overall sexual experience more pleasurable.

Unfortunately, some readers may want to disregard the advice given in this chapter. Such will be the fate of those who suffer back pain, and use that difficulty as an excuse for avoiding sexuality. Such people do exist. Pain problems are used for avoiding responsibilities and intimacy. Such avoidance techniques are the equivalent of statements used humorously, in common parlance, to describe the effect of pain on the ability to perform. The statement, "Not tonight dear, I have a backache," has meaningful connotations. Readers of this chapter may be either burdened or relieved to know that their chronic pain problems need *not* be a replacement for a fulfilling sexual life.

Epilogue: Some Parting Advice

Not long ago, I was rushing through the radiology department of the university hospital where I practice. I caught up to a colleague who specializes in cardiology, and we exchanged greetings. He then made a rather serious indictment of himself, which unfortunately applied even more accurately to me.

"I never cease to be astonished at the amount of sensible advice—about reducing their workload—that I give to my patients," he emphasized with remorse, "but that I totally disregard myself."

Although daily pressure and fatigue are not unique to the practice of medicine, I contemplated the rigors of having a conference scheduled at seven-thirty that morning and a staff meeting scheduled to last after nine that night. The intervening hours were to be overloaded with work. There would be patients scattered over numerous hospital wards, medical students and residents needing guidance, other medical specialists depending on my expertise as I depend on theirs, an office filled with harried people in distress, and an insatiable telephone. Hours full of pressure, of major and minor decisions, of facilitating health and relieving pain, of struggling to improve the quality and quantity of life.

Quite candidly, auto-acupressure provides the pain

relief which enables me to work that hectic schedule. Moreover, auto-acupressure is effective for my patients and also for my readers. Their letters of appreciation fill my file cabinets.

As I complete this epilogue in September 1979, I would like to share the contents of a letter which arrived this week. An attorney living in a distant state chronicled his battle with a pain problem, which lasted for a half-dozen years prior to acquiring my first book on auto-acupressure. He hoped that the promise of quick pain relief without drugs "might actually be realizable." He concluded:

> In 1977, I read about your book, bought it, read it and applied its principles. It works! The need for the "treatment" became less and less frequent and now a couple of weeks and more go by between symptoms. Upon auto-acupressure, they disappear in short order.
>   Your book has helped me tremendously and the virtual absence of pain has rekindled my enthusiasm for work. I am sure it has helped others—undoubtedly a lot more than you have heard from.

I must stress again that auto-acupressure for back pains is a medical, not a magical, technique. Many have felt that auto-acupressure has helped them recover from pain-related disabilities and enhanced their joy of life.

I hope you will share that experience.

Index

ABOUT THE AUTHOR

HOWARD D. KURLAND, M.D., is Professor, Department of Psychiatry at Northwestern University Medical School, and Senior Attending Psychiatrist, Evanston Hospital, Evanston, Illinois. He is past President of the Association for General Hospital Psychiatry, former Chief of Psychiatric Service of the Veterans Administration Research Hospital in Chicago, former Associate Professor of Neurology at Northwestern University Medical School and former Senior Attending Neurologist at Evanston Hospital. He is a Diplomate of the American Board of Psychiatry & Neurology and a Fellow of the Academy of Psychosomatic Medicine. He is a member of the Board of Directors of the Institute for the Advancement of Prosthetics, and past President of the Board of Directors of the National Board of Acupuncture Medicine.